Living with Cancer

Susan & Dennis
Wishing
you the
best

Vicly

Living
with
Cancer

A Step-by-Step Guide
....
for Coping Medically
....
and Emotionally
....
with a Serious Diagnosis

Vicki A. Jackson, MD, MPH
David P. Ryan, MD
with Michelle D. Seaton

Johns Hopkins University Press | Baltimore

Note to the reader: This book is not meant to substitute for medical care of people with cancer, and treatment should not be based solely on its contents. Instead, treatment must be developed in a dialogue between the individual and his or her physician. Our book has been written to help with that dialogue.

Drug dosage: The author and publisher have made reasonable efforts to determine that the selection of drugs discussed in this text conform to the practices of the general medical community. The medications described do not necessarily have specific approval by the US Food and Drug Administration for use in the diseases for which they are recommended. In view of ongoing research, changes in governmental regulation, and the constant flow of information relating to drug therapy and drug reactions, the reader is urged to check the package insert of each drug for any change in indications and dosage and for warnings and precautions. This is particularly important when the recommended agent is a new or infrequently used drug.

© 2017 Vicki Jackson and David Patrick Ryan
All rights reserved. Published 2017
Printed in the United States of America on acid-free paper
9 8 7 6 5 4 3 2 1

Johns Hopkins University Press
2715 North Charles Street
Baltimore, Maryland 21218-4363
www.press.jhu.edu

Library of Congress Cataloging-in-Publication Data

Names: Jackson, Vicki A., 1968–, author. | Ryan, David P., 1966–, author. | Seaton,
    Michelle D., author.
Title: Living with cancer : a step-by-step guide for coping medically and emotionally
    with a serious diagnosis / Vicki A. Jackson, MD, MPH, David P. Ryan, MD, Michelle D.
    Seaton.
Description: Baltimore : Johns Hopkins University Press, 2017. | Series: A Johns Hopkins
    Press health book | Includes index.
Identifiers: LCCN 2016033369 | ISBN 9781421422329 (hardcover : alk. paper) |
    ISBN 1421422328 (hardcover : alk. paper) | ISBN 9781421422336 (pbk. : alk.
    paper) | ISBN 1421422336 (pbk. : alk. paper) | ISBN 9781421422343 (electronic) |
    ISBN 1421422344 (electronic)
Subjects: LCSH: Cancer. | Cancer—Patients—Care. | Cancer—Psychological aspects. |
    Cancer—Patients—Life skills guides.
Classification: LCC RC263 .J33 2017 | DDC 616.99/4—dc23
    LC record available at https://lccn.loc.gov/2016033369

A catalog record for this book is available from the British Library.

Special discounts are available for bulk purchases of this book. For more information, please contact Special Sales at 410-516-6936 or specialsales@press.jhu.edu.

Johns Hopkins University Press uses environmentally friendly book materials, including recycled text paper that is composed of at least 30 percent post-consumer waste, whenever possible.

CONTENTS

Part III Dealing with Progressing Cancer

Every cancer specialist receives daily or weekly phone calls from friends of friends who have a cancer diagnosis or are in treatment and yet they have so many unanswered questions. These patients have all heard what the doctor said to them in the clinic—or thought they did—but afterward they often have trouble making sense of that information. This confusion is completely understandable. There are few experiences more disorienting than hearing the words, "You have cancer." Every phase of treatment can seem equally disorienting, like entering a new world filled with tests and scans and jargon. Patients are often at a loss as to how to ask the right questions of their oncologists and nurse practitioners about the treatments they undergo. They struggle to discuss in detail their emotions and symptoms in a busy clinical setting.

At Massachusetts General Hospital, we have come up with a novel integrated approach to treating patients with a serious cancer diagnosis. We offer them the opportunity to meet with both an oncologist and a palliative care specialist. The oncologist can focus on tests and scans and treatments for the cancer, while the palliative care specialist, with expertise in symptom management, focuses on how you are living with the cancer and the treatments. It's like meeting with an additional doctor, someone who is focused on how you are really doing, both physically and emotionally, living in this new cancer world.

For more than ten years, we have worked with many of the same patients, answering their questions while also offering each other our different perspectives on patient care. We've learned that it's not easy to stay oriented in the complex world of cancer treatment. People often need to hear information more than once. They need strategies to help them live fully and take advantage of the days when they feel strongest. And they love hearing about how other patients have dealt with situations similar to theirs. This book is the result of all of that work with our patients. We wanted to create a guide to help answer people's questions and empower them to ask many more questions of their own medical care team members.

When we decided to write this book, we enlisted the help of Michelle D. Seaton, a medical writer who was able to follow us in the clinic and watch our interactions with patients. She also interviewed patients and used all of this information to help craft our ideas into the book you hold now. Because of privacy concerns, the patient stories you read here are composites of the many thousands of patients we have treated.

This book reflects our understanding that the cancer experience is very different today than it was even a few years ago. New treatment options abound, including targeted therapies and better chemotherapy, which means that people who receive anticancer therapies often do well for a long time, even if their disease has spread beyond the original location (metastasized). We firmly believe that patients with a serious cancer diagnosis do better and feel better if they have a dedicated resource to help them manage the symptoms and side effects of treatment, one that motivates them to think about their goals, about the future, and about their quality of life. Patients feel more empowered when they have someone encouraging them to track and talk about their symptoms, someone who is offering them strategies for maintaining their quality of life. We wanted this book to be that resource. We want patients to concentrate on today, on living the best life they can right now.

Vicki A. Jackson, MD, MPH
David P. Ryan, MD

1

How Am I Going to Get through This?

VICKI ANSWERS FIRST:

I'm sorry that you have to read this book. This is probably the last place you thought you would be, reading a book about dealing with a diagnosis of cancer or helping someone you love adjust to this new reality. It can all feel surreal and overwhelming—the diagnosis, the medical jargon, the treatment options, the need to find specialists who can help you and with whom you feel comfortable. After a preliminary diagnosis, you may have a lot of urgent appointments for tests and further scans, or a biopsy or surgery, while also enduring days of anxious waiting. Throughout all of this it may seem impossible to believe any of the results. You want to shake the world and shout, "This can't be happening!"

It's hard for most medical professionals to fully understand the profound changes that people are asked to go through when they receive a cancer diagnosis. I got a glimpse of this shortly after I became a palliative care doctor. I remember standing in the lobby of a hospital in Boston on the morning of 9/11. We'd gathered there after news of a hijacking had spread, and we watched on TV as the towers collapsed. Like everyone else I kept watching it over and over again because I couldn't grasp what was going on. I saw it, but I couldn't quite believe it. That's when a patient took my arm and said, "That feeling you all have right now—that it's so unreal, that it can't be true. That's what it feels like to be told that you have cancer." I'm so grateful that he said that to me, because I now know that the first thing you have to get your mind around is how to understand that this is happening at all.

Very quickly, you have many more things to do as well. You have to build some kind of familiarity with your type of cancer and the obscure names of all the body parts affected by it. You have to learn to listen to an oncologist describing scans and lymph nodes and maybe the relative benefits of surgery, chemotherapy, and radiation. You have to figure out how to start a treatment regimen that will come with a long list of possible side effects. You have to find some context for your diagnosis and think about the future, knowing that it's going to be very different from what you had imagined. On top of that, you have to figure out how to keep living your life as normally as possible.

Having worked with thousands of patients who were dealing with a serious cancer diagnosis, I know that people need help with all of this. And I know that while Internet searches can sometimes be helpful, different websites can offer advice that is conflicting or even confusing. It's relatively easy to search for survival rates and treatment options; it's harder to figure out what these facts have to do with your situation. It's often bewildering to translate those facts into questions to ask your care team at various points in treatment.

That's why Dave and I wrote this book, to help guide patients and their family members through diagnosis and treatment, and to help them understand what has been said to them in their appointments and during chemotherapy treatments. Dave is a medical oncologist, and I'm a palliative care specialist. Together we've worked with thousands of patients, answering their questions about the likely course and outcome of their disease (prognosis) and treatment options, as well as helping them cope day to day. We have watched people go through this process and helped them get their bearings again. We've helped them feel confident and capable of getting through treatment while living their lives as fully as possible. Shortly after diagnosis, this may seem like an impossible goal, but you can do it. Armed with the right information, you can understand what each specialist is saying to you. You can make this less surreal. You can go on living your life.

This book grew from the professional relationship that Dave and I formed at Massachusetts General Hospital (MGH) in Boston. About fourteen years ago, the hospital created an outpatient palliative care program, designed to give cancer patients the chance to meet regularly with a specialist who works closely with their medical team. This doctor acts like a primary care physician for their cancer care, going over all of their prescriptions, addressing their side effects, asking about their emotional health and whether they need additional services to support them or their families.

At that time most oncologists referred patients to palliative care only at the end of life, to help them deal with the unique medical and emotional concerns that arise after anticancer treatments have been suspended. Some oncologists didn't understand how their patients would benefit from seeing an additional doctor or nurse practitioner earlier in treatment.

And yet when I met with patients, I found that I was sometimes the first person to ask them how they were spending their time every day, how they were sleeping, and whether there was something they wanted to do that they couldn't because of treatment. I also asked them detailed questions about how they were doing in the days after an infusion (intravenous chemotherapy) and went over all of the medications given to treat their symptoms, asking, "Is this working for you?" and, "How well is it working?" or, "Should we try something else?" Sometimes I found that patients were living with pain or constipation or other side effects that could be minimized with different medications, but they had not wanted to bring them up in the clinic. They wanted to put on a brave face for their oncologist. And that's normal. It's understandable. But my patients discovered that talking about their pain or nausea or anxiety and getting some help could change their lives. They could learn to track their symptoms and go into their appointment with a list and expect the medical team to address all of their concerns.

Some patients didn't know that they could tailor their treatments to minimize the disruption in their work schedules. Others didn't know that they could schedule a chemo holiday—a short break from treatment—to travel or attend a big family event. My hope is that this book will help you take control of your treatment.

The truth is that there is a gap between what traditional cancer care provides and what patients need. I don't blame oncologists for this. Medical oncology is an increasingly complex field. Every year brings more treatment options, new lines of chemotherapy, and new combinations of therapies. Top oncologists are busier than ever, and they have been taught to focus primarily on interventions that will kill cancer cells. It's what they have to do because the stakes are so high. And so the burden falls on patients and their family members to understand what's happening to their bodies and their lives.

During the first few years that I worked with cancer patients, there was little coordination between medical oncology and palliative care. Oncologists assumed that palliative care specialists didn't understand the virtues of chemotherapy and how much better patients feel when they have a great response to chemotherapy. And some palliative care specialists worried that oncologists were giving patients regimen after regimen of chemotherapy without paying enough attention to the side effects of treatment or the patient's quality of life. Neither of these assumptions was entirely correct, but they persisted. We had a lot to learn from each other. I had to learn about chemotherapy and how it worked and when it worked best. Oncologists had to learn how palliative care could help patients live better while they were receiving chemotherapy.

Many oncologists were slow to understand how to integrate this kind of care into their clinical practice, but Dave was an early proponent of palliative care. He understood what I was trying to do for patients in the cancer clinic. I hoped that if these two subspecialties could work together, we could create a powerful benefit for patients. We could make cancer treatment much more manageable for them. We could help them better understand a difficult prognosis and live their lives to the fullest while dealing with cancer.

Then Dave and I had a conversation one day that changed everything. It was about ten years ago, long before he had become the chief of hematology/oncology. At the time, he was a busy and well-respected GI (gastrointestinal) cancer specialist. That day I bumped into Dave in the cancer clinic and told him that I'd just met with one of his patients, a woman named Rebecca who had esophageal cancer. Her scans had come back showing that her cancer had grown through the first line of treatment. I clearly remember asking Dave what chemotherapy he would start her on next. Was he thinking about paclitaxel? He said yes, and I asked whether neuropathy (tingling or numbness in the hands and feet) was one of the common side effects. He said it was. I told him that Rebecca was already dealing with significant neuropathy from her first line of treatment. Was there another option? He later told me that he was stunned by this conversation, in part because Rebecca hadn't told him how much neuropathy she had been experiencing. I'll let him tell his side of the story.

I remember that conversation with Vicki really well. First, it was surprising to hear a palliative care doctor asking about a specific line of chemotherapy. Second, I was shocked that another doctor knew more about my patient's side effects than I did. I already knew that Vicki worked well with my patients, helping them cope with pain or other issues. Sometimes I would remind a patient that she'd had trouble with nausea after an infusion during our last visit and ask for more details, only to have the patient say, "Oh, I talked to Vicki about that. She took care of it." But this conversation about Rebecca's neuropathy had an impact on the regimen I chose for her, and it hinted at a much larger collaboration and how it could improve a patient's care.

It may be surprising to hear that a patient would keep a significant side effect secret from her doctor. After many years of working with palliative care, I've learned that it's actually not unusual for patients to be stoic about their side effects around their oncologists. Some people just want their oncology appointments to focus on treatments. Others don't know that their side effects could be better managed. A few people want to seem strong and capable to their oncologists, or perhaps they downplay unpleasant side effects because they don't want to disappoint their care team. People need help advocating for themselves when it comes to the issues that arise in the cancer setting. I've learned a lot from Vicki and from her team members about how to better help my patients manage these side effects so they can feel better and more like themselves day to day. I've learned to ask patients how they spend their time and what they want to be doing that they can't because of treatments. I've also learned how to better explain prognosis, and I don't worry if I have to explain these things more than once.

In the past ten years, outpatient palliative care has become a kind of mission at Mass General, specifically in the cancer clinic. Vicki has since become the chief of the Palliative Care Division at Mass General, and her team has grown more than 400 percent. Members of the oncology team, including nurses and nurse practitioners, have come to count on this palliative care perspective. We know that we are providing a singular level of care to patients coping with a difficult diagnosis, but at first this was just our belief. Then in 2010, my oncology colleague Jennifer Temel led a study looking at the effects of palliative care on patients with metastatic lung cancer (cancer that has spread to other parts of the body). In it, patients were offered standard treatment or standard treatment plus palliative care. At the end of the study, patients with palliative care lived on average 25 percent (almost three months) longer than did those with standard treatment alone. The study showed that patients who had a better understanding of their illness and a better quality of life spent less time in the hospital. They also expressed a far lower rate of depression than did patients with standard care alone. That study has been cited more than 2,500 times in the literature and it has lit a fire at major academic centers across the country. In 2012, the American Society of Clinical Oncology recommended that palliative care be systematically integrated in the care of all patients with metastatic solid tumors. The entire field of oncology has shifted as a result, and now many cancer centers are trying to integrate palliative care for their patients. I believe that this will become the new standard of care. As you can imagine, there are a lot of other studies under way that we hope will describe how this intervention works and which patients benefit the most.

Vicki and I wanted to write a book that wouldn't just describe the collaboration between palliative care and oncology but that would allow you to take advantage of everything that we've learned. Many patients don't yet have access to this kind of team approach, and yet they can benefit from what we know. Nearly every week, we get phone calls from friends of relatives who have a new diagnosis and so many questions. Why did the oncologist tell me this and what does it mean? What do I ask at my next appointment? When will we know if the treatment is working? Sometimes we get calls from distant friends with parents facing a difficult diagnosis. They ask what to do if the oncologist is recommending chemotherapy but their parent doesn't want it? How can they communicate their parent's wishes to the care team? Very few people have a friend of a friend who practices cancer care at a major teaching hospital. We wanted to tell readers what we tell people on the phone, and we want to talk to readers the same way we would talk to any friend, family member, or patient about the medical issues that arise with this kind of diagnosis. A lot of books confine themselves to describing one type of diagnosis, and it's true that every cancer is different when it comes to specific regimens or the latest clinical trials, but we've found that many patients face the same emotional concerns and many of the same medical issues, regardless of the type of cancer they are dealing with.

You won't need to read every chapter of this book. Not every patient has every symptom of cancer, and my hope and Vicki's is that you can turn to whatever chapters you need when you need them. Part I will take you through the initial stages of diagnosis and getting acclimated to treatment. Part II will help you troubleshoot any symptoms and side effects of treatment. Part III will talk you through what to expect and what to ask if your cancer continues to advance. Although many people won't need to read these last chapters, we have included several chapters on how to deal with end of life issues.

I've written the chapters in which the medical oncology perspective is most helpful. Vicki has written the chapters in which she can offer her palliative care expertise on matters such as coping with pain, nausea, weight loss, and other side effects, as well as coping emotionally. It's not important to focus on who has written any individual chapter. We want this book to show how this collaboration can give you the widest possible perspective on everything you may encounter in cancer treatment, regardless of your diagnosis.

Every year brings advances in the field of medical oncology. There are new treatments, including immunotherapy, and targeted therapies and newer lines of chemotherapy. While these treatments give more patients a much better chance at a cure, they also mean that more cancer patients are living longer with this diagnosis, even if the cancer can't be cured.

Vicki and I believe that patients need support while they learn to live well with cancer—to not merely endure treatments but to live fully for as long as they can. Many patients know at the time of diagnosis that their cancer isn't curable, but they find a way to live with their diagnosis, continuing to set goals for themselves, which may mean continuing to work or volunteer, or finishing a specific project or taking trips they've always dreamed about.

Let me give you an example.

Several years ago, a patient was referred to me because she'd had a mass in her abdomen that her doctors feared might be cancerous. When I met Susan, she was a forty-five-year-old attorney with two sons about to graduate from high school. That day she came to her medical appointment with a pathology report on a biopsy to sample the suspect tissue that had been done a couple of months before at a community hospital. She also had a list of physical symptoms that included flushing in the face and neck, diarrhea, and panic attacks. In that appointment Susan told me that she'd already been to four different oncologists, but she had not followed up with any of those doctors. The thought of being treated for cancer made it hard for her to breathe.

I immediately called Vicki to meet with Susan before our next appointment. It was Vicki who discovered that while Susan's panic attacks were related to her fear of cancer, her anxiety had been a lifelong problem. Vicki knew that she wanted to start treating the anxiety right away. She also explained to Susan what all of her oncologists had been telling her, including me: we didn't yet know whether the diagnosis was correct. Preliminary tests showed that she had some kind of cancer, but the biopsy was inconclusive. Vicki explained to Susan that she needed to find and stick to a treatment team and she needed more tests as soon as possible. She asked Susan whether she was willing to stay with my team for just one month so that more tests could be done.

Fortunately, Susan agreed, and even agreed to try some antianxiety medication in the short term. I arranged for an MRI (magnetic resonance imaging) scan and another biopsy, which showed Susan had neuroendocrine cancer that had started in her bowels and spread to the liver and lymph nodes. The tumor was producing serotonin, which was causing the flushing and diarrhea. Vicki started her on octreotide to counteract these symptoms and referred her to a psychologist, who could help with her anxiety. Vicki also helped Susan talk to her husband and children about her diagnosis. Unfortunately, cancer that has spread this far can't be cured. Both Vicki and I were able to give her family some context for this kind of cancer. They needed to know that some patients live years after this diagnosis, while others get sick quickly in the first couple of years.

Vicki's appointments with Susan were separate from mine, but Vicki and I spoke frequently about her progress. I worked with Susan on chemotherapy, scans, and testing, and Vicki worked with her on everything else she needed to know and do in order to live well with her diagnosis. This included scheduling treatments so that they didn't completely disrupt her law practice. It also meant setting personal goals for herself and doing things that were important to her in case the treatment didn't go as well as she hoped. In this book, we will explain how to do all of this. You will have the medical advice you need and the strategies for coping at every stage. Armed with this information, you can feel more in charge of your treatment and more able to deal with whatever happens.

Five years later, Susan is still coming to her appointments with Vicki and with me. The chemotherapy has worked well for her, and although she's needed a couple of surgeries in addition to her chemotherapy, her cancer is growing slowly enough that she has seen her children graduate from college. We still don't know how long she is going to live with cancer, but we do know that she is approaching her cancer in a methodical way. She is living well and enjoying her life.

Susan had an actual palliative care professional helping to explain the process of diagnosis and urging her to treat her most pressing symptoms right away. This book will help you do the same for yourself. It will walk you through your first appointment with an oncologist and tell you what to pay attention to in those early appointments and what questions to ask. It will explain how chemotherapy and radiation work, how to prepare for each, and how to make sense of whatever you learn about the possible trajectory of your illness. While in treatment, it will give you commonsense explanations for everything that might arise: from sudden infection to tricky bowel problems to dealing with fatigue, weight loss, or changes in sexual function. We will use a lot of patient stories, because we often tell these stories to our own patients. I think it's helpful, even comforting, to hear that other people have gone through these same experiences. You are not alone.

Vicki and I hope that you can use this book as an ongoing resource during treatment. You can think of it as a kind of field guide to the medical and emotional issues that often arise with a cancer diagnosis. We want you to have good information. We want to encourage you to ask more questions of your medical team so that you can get the best possible care, and also so that you can feel empowered and heard every step of the way. These are the most important things.

PART I

Making Sense of Your Diagnosis

2

Setting the Goals of Treatment

IF YOU HAVE A PRELIMINARY DIAGNOSIS of cancer and are still waiting for your first appointment with a medical oncologist, you may be wondering what that appointment is going to be like and how much information you are going to get. On the other hand, if you have already met with a medical oncologist, you may be wondering what happened, how to interpret all that you were told, and how to ask all the questions you still have. Patients sometimes complain that their first meeting with an oncologist is more rushed and businesslike than they were hoping. I can tell you that, from the oncologist's perspective, an initial appointment with a new patient is as tense as any first date. The stakes are very high, and it's really easy for doctor and patient to misread each other, to get off to an awkward start.

As a new patient, you also bring a lot of intense emotions to this appointment: hope, dismay, sadness, even anger. That's normal. And your oncologist is also anxiously trying to figure out what's going on based on your medical history and test results, and he or she is concerned about how to come up with the most successful treatment plan.

Sometimes patients think that they should concentrate on making sure the doctor knows them and their personal histories, so that the doctor will see them as a person rather than a patient. I love that idea, but like all oncologists I know that I'm going to get to know my patients well during the course of treatment. People choose to specialize in medical oncology because they like spending time with patients and because they want to help people who are dealing with a difficult diagnosis. So, in that first appointment, I'm trying to answer critical questions to get an accurate diagnostic picture and to make the right treatment plan for the patient.

There is a lot of ground to cover in this initial one-hour meeting. You will be asked many questions that may seem repetitive. At the same time, your oncologist is wondering about a number of issues while asking you all these questions and getting a medical history:

- *Do you have an actual diagnosis of cancer, or do we just think that there might be cancer?* Not every initial test is conclusive, and we can't start treatment until we know what we are treating. You might come to your first appointment thinking that you know you have cancer because a trusted doctor told you of his or her suspicions, but in oncology we say, "When tumor is the rumor, tissue is the issue." We trust a diagnosis of cancer only if a pathologist has viewed those cancer cells under the microscope.
- *What tests and scans will give us a better idea of the diagnosis?* If the tests and scans aren't conclusive, my first order of business is to figure out how we are going to make the actual diagnosis of cancer.
- *If you have an actual diagnosis of cancer, how secure am I with that diagnosis?* Does the diagnosis fit the picture shown by the pathology report, scans, and symptoms? Are we sure we know where the cancer started? Where the cancer starts is called the primary tumor. If we know where it started, we are better able to choose chemotherapy regimens that will be the most effective.
- *How far has the cancer advanced?* What kind of treatment plan would be best and how quickly do we need to start? Is surgery

a possibility? Might you need radiation in addition to chemo-therapy? Which specialists need to weigh in so that I'm sure you have the best chance at a cure, if that's possible, or so that you can live well for as long as possible?

The first visit may seem like a whirlwind, but that's because the oncologist is trying to gather enough information to answer these questions and then explain those answers to you. Remember that this is just the first visit. This is a lot of new and unsettling informa-tion to take in, and processing this information is an intensely per-sonal experience. As an oncologist, I know that while some people feel comfortable showing their emotions at such a time, others shut down or go quiet in order to protect themselves.

I know that some people are overwhelmed or angry or tuned out at some points during this first meeting as they try to take it all in. All of these reactions are common and normal. In fact, some people have very mixed feelings about their oncologist after the first appointment.

For example, I remember my first meeting with Phil, a sixty-five-year-old small business owner with a preliminary diagnosis of stage 4 colon cancer. I entered the exam room to find eight people there, including Phil and his wife, their three children, and their children's spouses. Phil runs a business in which he takes people on day-long fishing trips. The family had closed the business for the day to at-tend this appointment. That's how important it was to them. I took his medical history, went over the tests and scans, confirmed the di-agnosis of stage 4 colon cancer, and offered a treatment plan.

While the group had started out jovial and joking, they became silent as I talked about the diagnosis. I didn't know that they had come to this appointment desperately wanting this diagnosis to be a mistake and counting on me to say as much. When I finished talk-ing about treatment options, no one said a word. Phil didn't ask a single question. He stood, shook my hand, and they all left. I knew something had gone terribly wrong, but I didn't know what it was, and I didn't know whether I'd ever see Phil again. Fortunately, there are many great colon cancer specialists in Boston, and I knew he'd be in good hands if he went to someone else. I also knew that he was going to get the same diagnosis and the same treatment options from the next doctor he chose. For some people, it's easier to hear the diagnosis for the second time.

What surprised me was that Phil did come back for another appointment. He told me that his kids begged him to see someone else, someone who was more hopeful. But Phil told them that he liked me because I was straight with him. He has responded well to chemo and to surgery, and during the past several years I've gotten to know him and his family really well. Our appointments are completely different from that first encounter, always a lot of joking and laughing, and he still teases me about the fact that I was almost fired after that first one. For me, it's a great example of how awkward first meetings can be and how readily that tension fades once treatment begins.

The First Meeting with Your Oncologist

A lot is going to happen in your first meeting with an oncologist, and I think you'll have a better chance of staying oriented if you know what questions the doctor is likely to ask you before talking about your diagnosis, your pathology report, and the recommended treatment. The first half of every initial appointment is really a chance for the oncologist to gather significant information about your medical history. Yes, it can seem boring and repetitive, and, yes, you've already filled out lots of forms. Just keep breathing, and get through this first part, knowing that you will have more time to ask questions in the second half of the appointment.

Chief complaint. This is a fancy term for "what brings you here?" Sometimes doctors will send patients to an oncologist without fully explaining to them that they have cancer. It's critical for me to know why you think you're in my office. The oncologist will also ask for what's called a "history of present illness," which is a list of what symptoms you've experienced in the past few weeks and whether you've undergone any tests to reach a diagnosis.

Medications. Your doctor will want to know your current medications and doses, and if you have a list of them, it's good to bring it to the appointment. Your doctor will also ask whether you have any allergies to medications.

Medical history. You have probably filled out numerous forms detailing a lot of this, but the doctor will want to review them briefly as a way of keeping these details in mind as you go forward. This may be the point where you are thinking, "Can't we just get on with it? I want to know what the tests say." Believe me, the doctor knows how impatient you are.

Review of symptoms. The doctor will want to know how you are functioning in daily life. Are you sleeping? Are you in any pain? You may have to answer questions about your anxiety level, your bowels, your eating habits. Are there any activities that you can't engage in because of symptoms? Your doctor may want to help you relieve certain symptoms right away, even before your cancer treatment starts.

Physical exam. This is an opportunity for the doctor to look for any signs of the tumor in your body. Usually, this is brief, and often it's just a formality if we already know what we are going to find from the scans that you have had done. But your doctor wants to get every piece of information available.

Labs and scans. The doctor may review with you which blood tests and scans you've had done to make sure he or she has copies of all the information. I like to show people the scans if possible because it demystifies the cancer. The blobs and smears on the screen may not look like much to you, but they give a lot of information about the size of the tumors and how much the cancer has spread.

All of this should take place in the first half of your appointment. Don't be alarmed if the doctor seems to want to take in all of this information at a brisk pace. That's actually a good sign. Technically, this is a review of available information, but it's a necessary review. Some patients want to interrupt this process and chat, or they want to try to skip this part and get directly to the diagnosis and treatment plan. Your best strategy is to let the doctor ask all of these initial questions, answer them succinctly, and then be ready to take notes and ask a lot of questions when the doctor gets to the next part: going over the pathology report on your biopsy, giving you what doctors call the clinical picture. This is when your doctor discusses his or her impression—or diagnosis—and then recommends what kind of treatment would be best.

The Clinical Picture

Whenever one of my friends or family members goes to see an oncologist, I always tell them to spend the most time talking to the doctor about the pathology report and the stage of cancer. I know how hard that can be in the moment. Some people feel that the news is like a physical blow. Other people feel as though they are floating outside themselves, or they feel perfectly calm only to discover after the fact that they have only hazy memories about the entire medical visit. Almost every week, I get a phone call from a friend of a friend asking me for advice about a first appointment with an oncologist. It's hard to give advice when the person on the other end of the phone can't remember anything about the stage of cancer or the test results. Then it becomes a guessing game. Did the doctor talk about lymph nodes? How about metastases? Did the doctor talk about the size of the tumor or the margins? I sometimes ask these people to read the pathology report to me over the phone, because it contains details about the cancer cells, tumor size, and how far the cancer is spread, and this information will be the foundation for what the oncologist suggests as treatment options. You can and should get a copy of the pathology report at this first meeting.

That's why I also tell people to bring a notebook or a recording device to this first meeting. It's great to have another person in the room, so you can double the chances that you walk away knowing the staging and the pathology report. These are the crucial pieces of information to listen to, to ask questions about, and to remember later. When your doctor communicates with other specialists about you, he or she will likely refer primarily to these two things.

So, first, let's look at what's likely to be in your pathology report.

The Pathology Report

When tissue has been taken from someone's body because a doctor suspects cancer, a pathologist takes that tissue and examines it under a microscope. The tissue can come from a biopsy, which is a sample of cells taken from a suspected tumor, or it can come from a surgeon who has removed all or part of the tumor. If your doctor suspects a liquid tumor (discussed in chapter 4), such as leukemia or lymphoma, your biopsy may have been taken from your blood or bone marrow. After examining the tissue sample or the entire tumor, the pathologist will fill out a report with the following information: diagnosis, tumor size and grade, margins, immunohistochemistry, and molecular pathology and genotyping.

Diagnosis. The pathologist will categorize the type of cancer cell found in the tumor or sample. Types include:

- adenocarcinoma, a broad term for cancers that arise in duct-forming organs like the breast, lung, colon, and pancreas;
- squamous cell cancer, the broad term for cancers that can appear in the skin, mouth, head and neck, anus, cervix, and vagina;
- melanoma, a type of cancer that develops in the skin;
- sarcoma, cancer cells that can develop in muscle and bone;
- leukemia or lymphoma, cancer cells that develop in the blood or lymphatic system.

Sometimes, the pathologist can state definitively what type of cell is in the sample, which helps doctors figure out the organ in which the cancer started, if it's a solid tumor. This diagnosis is the cornerstone of everything that will happen in treatment, so be sure to ask your oncologist whether this diagnosis is straightforward and definitive. If it's not, you may want to ask for a second opinion from another pathologist.

Tumor size. If an entire tumor was removed, the pathologist will measure it from several angles and record the largest measurement as the tumor size. Sometimes the size of the tumor matters, and, as you might imagine, the smaller the tumor, the better. But you should ask your oncologist whether the size of the tumor matters in your case. Tumor size often isn't relevant if you have leukemia or lymphoma or some cancers in the gastrointestinal system.

Tumor grade. This tells us how aggressive the cancer looks under the microscope. In some cancers, this is not relevant, but in other cancers, such as lymphomas, it is a critical piece of information.

Margins. Again, if an entire tumor has been removed, the surgeon will also have removed some of the normal tissue surrounding the tumor, so that it can be examined for the presence of cancer cells. The result of this examination is crucial. I often give patients the example of a jellyfish. You can see the red center of the jellyfish but you always give it a wide berth because you know it has tentacles that you can't see. A negative margin or a clear margin indicates that the surgeon removed the visible tumor as well as those tentacles of tumor that were not visible. That's what the surgeon means (or hopes) when he or she says, "We got it all."

A positive margin can mean that there was more cancer in the area than the surgeon could see. It also means that the cancer is much more invasive and therefore less likely to be curable. Usually, you don't need a second opinion on tumor margins because the original pathologist is the only person who knows how the tumor was laid out and how much tissue the surgeon took out. A close margin usually means that the tumor came within millimeters of where the surgeon cut. Close margins are usually associated with a higher risk of the cancer coming back locally. The status of the margin is another factor that won't matter if you have a liquid tumor, such as leukemia or lymphoma.

Immunohistochemistry. Pathologists can stain tissues with substances that reveal more characteristics about the cancer cells. This process can detect certain cell markers that can give more information about the likely prognosis and give clues about how the cells may respond to treatment. The relevant question to ask is whether the immunohistochemistry is consistent with the diagnosis. If it's not, ask why not. This is where a second opinion on the pathology might be appropriate.

Molecular pathology and genotyping. The genetics of the tumor are becoming a more significant part of the pathology report. However, we have to wait several weeks or even months for the full genotyping to be done. In this report, pathologists determine which mutations and gene alterations occurred in your tumor. This is not the same as inheriting a predisposition to cancer. This part of the report usually describes how the DNA of your tumor has changed from the DNA of normal tissue to become a cancer.

Here's a quick primer on DNA, which stands for deoxyribonucleic acid. It is the building block of our entire body. DNA gets translated in the cell into RNA (ribonucleic acid). RNA in turn gets translated into proteins. Proteins are the building blocks of the cell or the pistons in the engine. All you really need to know is that it's the over-expression of some proteins and the underexpression of other proteins that leads to a cancer.

Sometimes, this information can lead to significant treatment changes. It is extremely important that you ask your oncologist whether molecular pathology or genotyping is significant in your type of cancer.

Tests and Scans That Help with Staging

The second most important thing to pay attention to in this meeting is the stage of your cancer. If your doctor is able to stage your cancer in this first meeting, that's probably because you've had one or more scans that allow doctors to look at the rough outlines of the tumor and study its exact location. Your doctor may have ordered additional scans of your whole body or other parts of your body to search for metastases, or small tumors that may be visible in other areas of the body. This information, combined with notes from the surgeon and the pathology report of the biopsy or tumor will provide the information needed to set the stage of your cancer.

You should get information about staging at your first appointment with your medical oncologist, unless more testing needs to be done. (We talk more fully about tests and scans in chapter 6.) At a major teaching hospital, there is a whole system in place for staging cancer, so at the first suspicion of cancer, the patient will meet with an interventional radiologist or surgeon who will order scans and then do a biopsy for the pathologist. These are the details doctors need to give you staging information. At smaller community hospitals, the medical oncologist is often responsible for ordering those tests and then making the diagnosis.

What Is the Stage of My Cancer?

You may already know that all cancers have four stages—except for some hematologic malignancies and brain tumors, which are staged differently (hematologic malignancies, or cancers of the blood, are discussed in chapter 4). For every other type of cancer, we talk about stages in terms of the numbers 1 through 4. This is an internationally recognized staging process for all cancer established by the World Health Organization.

- *Stage* 1. Cancer that is small and localized, meaning it hasn't spread anywhere, and is usually curable.
- *Stages 2 and* 3. Cancer that has advanced either to lymph nodes or to tissue surrounding the tumor or the organ of origin. These cancers often require chemotherapy and radiation in addition to surgery to be cured, but they are often curable. I've lumped these two stages together because, in some cancers, the difference between stage 2 and stage 3 is trivial. In other types of cancer the difference is enormous in terms of how the oncologist will want to treat it and how likely it is that the cancer will continue to spread despite treatment.
- *Stage* 4. This is cancer that has spread beyond the original tumor location, beyond the surrounding lymph nodes, and has likely settled in other areas of the body. Stage 4 cancers, except for lymphomas, are usually not curable.

Am I Curable?

You do want to ask this question after your doctor has staged your cancer, but I will warn you that the doctor might not have a definitive answer. Usually when doctors talk about being cured, we mean that after treatment the cancer is gone and doesn't come back even after five years. But this isn't always the case, because some cancers do return. You can follow up by asking what the chances are that you might be cured. This is where you want to ask a lot of questions about the type of treatment the oncologist is suggesting and how likely you are to be cured if you agree to all of these treatments.

Sometimes it's clear that a cancer should be curable. For example, a relatively small tumor that has not spread to the lymph nodes or any other areas usually has a good chance of being cured. I remember one patient who came to me about ten years ago with a diagnosis of stomach cancer. She was relatively young, but her mother had died of stomach cancer at a similar age, so this patient assumed that she would also die. In fact, she was already getting her affairs in order, and her main treatment questions were about managing pain. I had to say to her, "No, I think we can cure this." She didn't quite believe me at first, but her cancer was curable. I still hear from her sometimes.

However, if the cancer has spread into the liver and other organs, it's likely not curable. But in some cases there's a possibility of cure with aggressive treatment, and in that case you want to ask how aggressive the treatment has to be to give you that chance.

The Goal of Treatment

The first question you want to ask after staging is what the oncologist hopes treatment will do for you. By knowing the goal of treatment, you can better choose treatment options that are right for you. We can talk about the goal of treatment only when we know the pathology and the staging. I've had patients blurt out in the first several seconds that they are never going to do chemotherapy, before they even know the diagnosis, stage, and treatment options. Or I've had patients say that they will do everything to fight the cancer and try to beat it. People and the media always talk about fighting cancer, but oncologists don't think in these terms. We think in terms of the goals of treatment. There are just three possible goals in treatment:

1. *Cure the cancer.* This means using the standard treatments of surgery, radiation, and chemotherapy to kill or remove the cancer cells from your body.
2. *Prolong your life.* If your type of cancer can't be cured, your doctor may recommend these same standard treatments in the hope of giving you as much time as possible. Even when cancer can't be cured, it can often be controlled, meaning the growth of tumors can be slowed down, so that you will live longer.
3. *Make you feel better.* Even when your doctor knows that treatments won't cure you or prolong your life, he or she may recommend treatments that will make you much more comfortable.

Nothing should be prescribed for you unless it fits one of these stated goals: to try to cure the cancer, to prolong life, or to make you feel better. And this is a good time to ask your doctor what the goals of treatment are. What does your doctor think is possible for you? You also want to be thinking about your goals and values. How much treatment do you want? How aggressive can those treatments be while allowing you to maintain your quality of life?

Your Goals and Values

Sometimes the goal of therapy changes when people find out what it will take to have a chance at a cure. I'm treating an author who lives in the Berkshires and has metastatic colon cancer. We talked about how surgery alone would be unlikely to cure her cancer and that if she had additional chemotherapy and radiation, her likelihood of a cure would go up by about 10 percent. It was going to be a tough treatment regimen, one that would likely have disrupted her work life, making it impossible to finish her novel. She told me that she was perfectly comfortable with surgery alone because finishing her novel meant more to her than gaining a better chance of surviving the cancer. So her goal changed. Instead of pursuing the chance of a cure at all costs, she decided to forego chemotherapy because she believed that the treatment wasn't worth the better odds it offered for a cure.

If the doctor tells you that your cancer isn't curable, you still have choices about what treatments to use to control the cancer. Surgery, chemotherapy, and radiation treatments are all disruptive, and you will need to think about what you want to endure to prolong your life. Some people view living as long as they possibly can as the ultimate goal, while others prefer to emphasize living as well as they can. For example, one of my patients has a slow-growing gastrointestinal stromal tumor, and the recommended treatment includes imatinib to help slow the tumor's growth. Even though this medication is working as it should and keeping the tumor growth down, it has side effects that that patient hates. As a result, she insists upon taking treatment breaks that may shorten her life. She has decided that gaining extra time, even if it's a year or two, isn't worth the side effects of continuous treatment.

Even if the goal of treatment is to make you comfortable, you have choices about which treatments you do and don't want. You can opt for some disease-modifying treatments to pursue that goal. For instance, I had a patient who told me that she didn't want to do anything except see Vicki in palliative care to manage the symptoms and side effects of her cancer, because she didn't want any more chemotherapy. She later developed a small metastasis in her rib right underneath her armpit. Every time she rolled over in her sleep a sharp jab of pain would wake her up. She experimented with all types of pain and sleeping medicines, but nothing worked. I finally convinced her to let us radiate the rib metastasis. After three short treatments the next week, she started to notice improvement. She was sleeping through the night without any pain two weeks after the radiation finished.

Knowing the goal of treatment as well as your values empowers you throughout treatment. It gives you the ability to choose treatments that help you achieve your goal and to refuse treatments that you don't want. Early on, you may want to pursue every treatment to have a chance at curing a cancer or to prolong your life. Over time, that goal may change, and that's okay.

The Treatment Plan

Once your doctor tells you what your type of cancer is and the stage, he or she may talk about a plan for treatment. Just as there are only three goals of cancer treatment (cure, live longer, feel better), there are only three broad options to treat a cancer:

- *Standard therapy*, using recognized, proven therapies studied by oncologists, designed to eradicate the cancer or keep it in check for as long as possible.
- *Experimental therapy*, which involves clinical trials. Some clinical trials may involve newer, less-proven therapies, while other clinical trials are evaluating standard regimens.
- *Supportive care alone*, which will keep you comfortable and active for as long as possible or simply monitor for the possible recurrence of cancer.

That's it. I always give people treatment options in all three categories, but I also initiate a conversation about the patient's goals and values and then make a recommendation for treatment based on that. Some oncologists offer a lot of treatment options as though it's an à la carte menu and then ask you to choose the best option. And while I agree that the patient ultimately decides on the treatment option, I disagree with the à la carte menu approach. Patients should make treatment decisions in line with their values. You have the right to choose whether you want to undergo a specific type of treatment. I've had patients who have come out of surgery with clear margins and good prognosis to whom I have recommended chemotherapy because it improves their chance of being cured and because that's what I would have chosen for myself. And in some cases patients have said, "No, thanks." Some patients know exactly what they want and don't want, and I respect that.

But I also know that some people struggle with the burden of choosing treatment. The last thing I want patients to feel is that they are all alone in making this decision.

For example, seventy-eight-year-old Margaret is a retired lawyer who has stage 3 colon cancer. She has three options. We can pursue supportive care alone in which we will help her recover from her surgery and follow her closely for recurrence. She has a 75 percent chance of being cured without any chemotherapy. She could choose to pursue standard chemotherapy for six months, which will improve her chances of being cured to 80 percent. And finally, we have an experimental clinical trial for patients with stage 3 colon cancer in which we add a drug to the standard regimen. We don't know that the drug in this clinical trial is any better or worse than standard chemotherapy. It could be better than standard treatment. In fact, it could become the new standard of treatment in five years. But we don't know that.

Margaret's number one fear is that she won't be around to take care of her husband, who has just been diagnosed with Alzheimer's. She would feel awful if she didn't do everything possible to be around for him. But she needs to have all her strength to help him now, and she believes the clinical trial with its extra visits and extra chances of side effects is not the right choice. So we make a decision together to give her six months of chemotherapy to give her the best chance possible to be cured.

Can I Die from Treatment?

The final question you want to ask is a tough one. Ask whether there is a chance that certain side effects are permanent or whether there is a chance that you could die from a side effect of treatment. For many standard chemotherapy treatments, there is a 0.5 to 1 percent chance of dying from the treatment. While it's not high, it's not as low as for other medications. This is a meaningful discussion to have with your oncologist, particularly if you have other chronic health issues. Nobody likes to think about the possibility of dying from treatment, but some treatments do come with a higher risk of death, and you want to have this information before you begin.

For example, I had a patient who was diagnosed with pancreatic cancer. Charlie was seventy-nine years old at the time of diagnosis, and he was also coping with diabetes, mild kidney dysfunction, and heart failure. I explained to Charlie that he could have the tumor removed with surgery and then undergo chemotherapy for a chance at a cure, but that the treatments came with a lot of risk. Charlie's wife asked the critical question, which was how likely was he to die if he had the surgery, given his other medical issues. The answer was that he had a 10 to 20 percent chance of dying in surgery. Although Charlie was optimistic about his chances, he and his wife agreed to think about this more and talk to their children before deciding on a course of treatment.

Oncologic Emergencies

Even at this early stage of diagnosis for cancer, emergencies can occur. At any time in your treatment, if you experience the following symptoms, call your doctor or the clinic immediately, regardless of the time. In the following instances (table 2.1), you want a call back from a clinician within ten to fifteen minutes. If you don't hear back from a clinician and are feeling unwell, you should go to the emergency room.

Fever greater than 100.5 degrees Fahrenheit (38 degrees Celsius) in the setting of chemotherapy	Might indicate low white blood cell count (febrile neutropenia) and the need for antibiotics
Fever greater than 100.5 degrees Fahrenheit (38 degrees Celsius) and shaking chills	Might indicate bacteria in the bloodstream
New confusion	Might indicate brain metastasis or serious side effects from medications
Back pain with neurologic symptoms (leg weakness or rubberiness; difficulty holding bladder or bowels)	Might indicate spinal cord compression
Swelling of the neck and face with distended veins	Might indicate the main veins in the neck are blocked (superior vena cava syndrome)
Coughing up blood	Might indicate bleeding into the lung
More than a teaspoon of bright red blood in the toilet	Might indicate gastrointestinal bleeding
Black tarry stools (particularly if not taking supplemental iron)	Might indicate gastrointestinal bleeding
Acute chest pain particularly when taking in a deep breath with or without shortness of breath	Might indicate a blood clot in the lungs (pulmonary embolus)

Choosing a New Oncologist

Often I hear from friends who live in another part of the country and who are dealing with a cancer diagnosis for themselves or a loved one. And they want to know how to find the best oncologist, or they want to fire the oncologist they have and find a new one. I tell them to look for someone who has treated a lot of people with your type of cancer. Some people want a doctor who is prominent in the field, but that's not as important as finding someone who is a good communicator.

One of my colleagues uses what he calls the 3 A's for judging a doctor: able, available, and affable. By that, he means that your oncologist's first responsibility is to be competent in his or her specialty. Second, a great doctor is available to patients. You want to have a phone number that you can call at any time and know that the doctor or nurse practitioner will get back to you quickly. The third marker for greatness in a doctor—affability—is harder to come by among oncologists. A few oncologists are charming, but many great oncologists tend to be more serious or a bit shy. So affability for an oncologist may mean finding someone who can explain technical issues and options and who is emotionally supportive.

You want to work with a doctor who invites questions and answers them, someone who sees you as a person, someone you can call at any time, someone you trust. When you are getting references, be sure to ask about the doctor's communication style. When you meet with a new doctor, be sure to ask, "How can I reach you if I need something?" You also want to work with someone who is part of a well-staffed team, so that there are nurse practitioners, nurses, social workers, and other team members who can talk to you any time and see you right away when you need advice and help.

3

Understanding the Biology of Cancer

TO UNDERSTAND WHAT YOUR FUTURE may be like with cancer, you might want to understand how cancer cells are different from normal cells and how cancer spreads. You might want to know what your stage of cancer means for the goals of treatment, and under what circumstances your staging might change. For some people, having a lot of information helps them cope with all of the changes treatment brings and helps them make plans for the future, specifically, how to think about what might happen if treatment doesn't work as well as we all hope.

Not everyone wants to read about the spread of cancer or know all about what staging means. And you don't have to read this chapter at all in order to go through treatment or to live well with cancer. You can read this information now if you feel ready, or save it for later. Vicki and I often tell people that it takes at least three months to get your mind around the idea that you are being treated for cancer. And after that adjustment period, you may be better able to think about and talk to your oncologist about the future. For some people it takes even longer, and that's fine, too.

For example, I have a patient who was diagnosed with a pancreatic endocrine tumor. (This is far different from pancreatic cancer, which is an adenocarcinoma of the pancreas and can be very aggressive.) At the time of diagnosis, Daphne was fifty-three years old and the chief financial officer of an insurance company. She underwent successful surgery to remove the tumor, but because we'd determined that she was at stage 3, the likelihood was high that the cancer would return.

Daphne and I had long discussions about the nature of endocrine tumors. I explained in detail how cancer spreads and why I was so concerned about a recurrence. She always smiled and nodded while I talked, and I was completely amazed by her calm demeanor. It was as though nothing could shake her. Only later did she tell me that she wasn't listening to me during any of those appointments. Instead, she was counting backward from a hundred by increments of three, a trick she'd learned to keep herself calm during heated meetings at work. "I didn't have time for cancer," she said, admitting that she couldn't think about her prognosis (the likely course and outcome of her disease) rationally for the first six months. She couldn't even bring herself to tell her college-aged children while she was still trying to understand it herself. Fortunately, her type of cancer has been slow growing, so by the time we did detect another tumor in her liver—meaning that it had become metastatic—she was ready to really listen to all of this information. She has had the cancer now for more than ten years and has retired and travels with her husband.

The Scope of Cancer

It can be extremely frustrating to hear your doctor refer to your chances at a cure or to refer to the chances that your cancer might recur. You may be wondering, Why are there so many statistics and so few definitive answers? Why are we talking about my life as though it's a lottery?

Doctors aren't using this kind of language to be cagey. They are talking in terms of percentages because they know that it is impossible to measure the actual scope of cancer in someone's body.

Tumors grow because the cells in them are constantly dividing, but they also shed cells that can circulate either in the bloodstream or the lymph nodes. Most of these won't seed other tumors, but a few of them might. They can get caught in the tissues of other organs, such as the liver or lungs, and start dividing again. If these cells have seeded a new tumor in the same area from which it was originally removed, we call it a local recurrence. If the cells have traveled to another part of the body, we call it a systemic recurrence.

Unfortunately, cancer cells can grow and accumulate long before scans can detect them. In fact, a tumor has to be close to one centimeter in size, about the size of a marble, before it can be detected on a scan. And that single, small tumor can contain close to a billion cancer cells. If you have a cluster of cancer cells nearby or in another organ and that cluster contains only one hundred million cells, we probably can't yet see it.

How Cancer Spreads

Cancer is a disorder of genes, which means that the DNA that encodes the genes of a specific cell has mutated. Of course, cells are acquiring mutations all the time as individual cells divide. Some mutations you have inherited, and some you have acquired just by being alive. But sometimes cells can acquire enough mutations in specific parts of the genes that control the cell's growth to cause these cells to replicate out of control. They don't behave like normal cells in that they don't die naturally as other cells are programmed to do. Sometimes, your immune system will target these cells and kill them. But if you have cancer, the immune system response has failed to kill these cells. It doesn't mean that something is wrong with your immune system. It just means that the cancer has figured out how to evade your immune cells. If the cancerous cells continue to grow and mutate, they may gain the ability to move through natural barriers, such as the membranes that divide cells and tissues, and then spread through the bloodstream. So, cancer cells are sort of like supercells that grow despite all your body's best efforts to stop them.

Also, your cancer cells are unique to you. No two cancers will have exactly the same mutations, and that's why your cancer cells will be slightly different from the cancer cells of every other patient you meet, even if you both have a similar diagnosis.

So, when your doctor says that there is a chance at a cure or a chance of recurrence, he or she is basing those percentages on all the accumulated research on your type of cancer. In fact, this system for classifying solid tumors is called the TNM staging system. The letters stand for tumor, node, and metastases.

TNM Staging System

This is a straightforward system for classifying solid tumors and describing how the cells in them have behaved so far in the system. (For hematologic cancers, or cancers of the blood, see chapter 4.)

The "T" represents the size of the tumor, and it gets a classification from 1 to 4. Generally, a T1 tumor is small and a T4 tumor is large, although a tumor can have a higher number if it has invaded tissue just outside the place of origin. If a tumor is large, there is a higher likelihood that it has seeded other tumors in the same organ or in other areas of the body.

Lymph nodes near the tumor may also contain cancer cells, which is described by the "N." Your doctor may describe your cancer as node negative (or N0) if there is no cancer in the lymph nodes. If nodes do show some cancer cells, they are called node positive (or N1). Sometimes cancers are further described by the number of nodes that are involved, so you can get numbers such as N2. Of course, the more nodes that are involved, the more likely it is that the cancer has taken root elsewhere.

We use the letter "M" to describe metastases, which is the presence of cancer at a site different from where the cancer started. So, if you have colon cancer but there are also small tumors in the liver, these liver tumors are metastases, which doctors and nurses sometimes call "mets." If you have metastases, your cancer will be described as M1, and if not, it will be called M0.

Some people think that when the cancer appears in another part of the body, it is a different kind of cancer, but it's not. Lung cancer is always lung cancer, even if it spreads to the bones or liver. Sometimes I tell patients that I grew up in New York as a Mets fan, and even though

I've moved to Boston, I still describe myself as a Mets fan. If I move to Texas, I will still be a Mets fan. Your cancer cells are the same in that no matter where they go in your body we still describe them as the same type of cancer based on where the cells originated.

When your doctor puts together the TNM numbers, he or she will know your stage of cancer. You should always know your TNM stage because it is a much more precise description of your cancer at the time of diagnosis and because this staging will determine how your medical team wants to treat the cancer. Your oncologist will always remember your TNM stage at diagnosis. It is probably the one thing your doctor will remember about you when you bump into her in the grocery store in ten years. You can look up the TNM numbers on one of any number of charts on the Internet and find out the more general stage (such as stage 1 or stage 3).

Is My Cancer Curable?

The discussion about whether your cancer is curable is one of the toughest conversations you will have with your oncologist. As chief of hematology/oncology, I'm often asked by colleagues and friends to advise their family members who have just been diagnosed with metastatic disease. When I speak to them, I find that many have been devastated by the news that their cancer is not curable. In fact, they may not have paid much attention to anything else that was said to them in that first meeting with their oncologist. They may not remember their stage or diagnosis, and they sometimes don't know what the treatment plan might be. It may take days to begin to comprehend that your life has been changed by a cancer diagnosis. And it can be confusing to try to think about possible treatment options in the moments after your doctor has given you the news. You may have found yourself feeling angry at the doctor for the way he or she explained your diagnosis or worried for family members who depend on you, or you may have jumped ahead, as many patients do, to ask, "How long do I have?" All of these are normal reactions.

Whenever I'm advising a friend of a friend about how to understand a diagnosis, I always give him or her specific questions to ask the oncologist during the next visit. The answers to these questions will help frame the conversation so you can better understand what's going on. The answers your doctor gives to these questions will help guide you down the path that's best for you. These questions are about the best-case and worst-case scenarios for your type of cancer. You should always ask these questions:

- What is the best-case scenario for treatment?
- How likely is that to happen?
- What do I have to do to give myself the best chance at a best-case scenario?
- How long will I have to go through treatment to get a chance at a best-case scenario?
- Is it worth it?
- What is a worst-case scenario for my type of cancer?
- What is the most likely scenario?

What Is My Best-Case Scenario?

Your doctor's goal is to give you the best chance at a best-case scenario. That might be a cure, or it might be to live well for several more years. Sometimes the best-case scenario requires no further work on your part. Many early-stage cancers don't require you to do anything more than follow up with your oncologist at regular intervals. Even if you have metastatic cancer, the best-case scenario is often measured in years, sometimes many years.

It's important to talk about what kind of treatment is required to give you your best-case scenario, because treatment might require trade-offs that you are not willing to make. Lilliana is a sixty-eight-year-old woman with stage 4 rectal cancer that might be curable. To pursue a cure, she would need to undergo at least two major operations, six months of chemotherapy, and then radiation therapy. At the end of all of that, she would have about a 10 percent chance of being cured. She decided that she wasn't willing to make those trade-offs. I've had a lot of other patients facing the same odds who really did want to pursue treatment with the hope of being cured.

What Is My Worst-Case Scenario?

This is a tricky question because not everyone would define the worst outcome in the same way. Many oncologists will define the worst outcome as dying in the first year after diagnosis; some, the first six months. That can happen if the cancer treatment doesn't work as well as we hope or if the patient experiences a complication during treatment. Some people may not want to talk or even think about that possibility, but it is important to ask about it, even if you don't want to think about it ever again and just want to focus on treatment.

I also get a lot of calls from friends whose older parents have been diagnosed with late-stage cancer and don't know what kind of treatment, if any, that mom or dad will want. One friend called recently to say that her mother had been diagnosed with pancreatic cancer and that the oncologist was pushing to start chemotherapy right away. But my friend's mother was in her mideighties and wasn't sure she wanted to endure that. I helped my friend talk through the questions of best-case and worst-case scenarios with her mom's oncologist, and the oncologist told her that the best-case scenario would be that her mom would live for a year. But to achieve that, she would have to undergo a very aggressive chemotherapy regimen that would significantly alter her quality of life. When asked, my friend's mother said that there was no way she wanted to go through that. And although my friend was sad, she agreed that the treatments would be too difficult for her mom. The worst-case scenario would be that her mom would die in one to two months. But with appropriate medical supervision and with the aid of hospice, her mother could expect to live at home, where she could spend time with family, and then to die at home. The goal of therapy then became how to best support her medically in the time she had left. This is when family can really support a patient and work with a medical team to make sure everybody understands the patient's goals for treatment.

Survival Rates

It can be unsettling to look at survival rates for your type and stage of cancer, even in the best circumstances. Many patients look them up online after the initial diagnosis, although you don't have to do this. Some people check them immediately, while others refuse to look at them. Most survival statistics report both the five-year and the average survival rate. The problem with these statistics is that they don't take into account specific issues that will affect the prognosis, such as other medical problems and overall health. Also, finding out that an average survival rate for a certain type of cancer is 60 percent after five years is unhelpful at best. That's why I tend to talk to patients about best-case and worst-case scenarios. Everything depends on the biology of the tumor and the way that your cancer responds to standard treatment.

Also, the statistics themselves can be misleading. You are a person, not a statistic, and your cancer cells are unique to you. Early in my career I worked with two patients whose experiences with cancer were the opposite of what the statistics indicated. Melissa had a stage 1 colon cancer and a 90 percent chance of being alive in five years, and I told her so. JoAnn had stage 4 colon cancer and the survival statistics indicated that she had a 10 percent chance of being alive in five years. That was a difficult discussion, but I believe that doctors should talk to patients about what might happen if the treatments don't work as well as we hope. I was thrilled when JoAnn's cancer responded wonderfully to therapy, and even happier when she underwent surgery and had the tumor removed.

Five years later, JoAnn scolded me, saying that I should never tell anyone their survival statistics. She said that she had lived in terror during that first year, thinking that each holiday and family birthday would be her last. Melissa wasn't so fortunate. Despite having a very hopeful survival statistic, her cancer returned in the fourth year after treatment. It became clear that the cancer had spread. She told me that I should have warned her more strongly that this was a possibility. She said she would have lived differently if she had realized that time was so short.

Doctors can't be completely accurate when they provide prognostic estimates. Every oncologist has had patients like Melissa and JoAnn, who have had outcomes that did not follow statistical predictions. That's why some doctors are so uncomfortable talking about prognosis.

I hope you can have some kind of conversation with your oncologist about the possible trajectory of your illness. That doesn't mean you have to be aware of your best- and worst-case scenarios every minute. It doesn't even mean that your prognosis is correct. When Vicki works with patients, she sometimes asks them to talk about what they hope for in treatment and what they worry about the most. This is a terrific tool for understanding your illness. You can even use this technique on your oncologist, if he or she doesn't like to talk about prognosis. You can ask what the oncologist hopes will be the result of treatment, and what he or she is worried might happen.

Chance of Recurrence

If your cancer is stage 1 to stage 3, and potentially curable or likely curable, your doctor will talk to you about the chance that the cancer might recur even if the treatment is successful. For patients with stage 2 or stage 3 cancer, there can be a substantial risk of the cancer returning. You may know someone who had a surgery to remove a tumor and then some years later the cancer came back. Of course, the cancer didn't exactly return. Technically, the cancer cells were hiding somewhere else in the body and then took hold and grew into additional tumors. For some types of cancer, the risk of recurrence is as high as 90 percent, but for others it is much lower, such as 20 percent. During these discussions, patients sometimes ask whether there is anything else they can do to give themselves a better chance at being completely cured. That's when we have a long discussion about adjuvant chemotherapy. The word "adjuvant" comes from the Latin word *adjuvare*, and it means "to aid" or "to help." Adjuvant chemotherapy or radiation given after surgery helps people to be cured more often than they would if they had surgery alone. Sometimes we offer these treatments before surgery, and then we call it neoadjuvant, or preoperative, therapy. By using chemotherapy or radiation, we are trying to eliminate those cancer cells that may be hiding.

Adjuvant Treatment

It can be confusing to understand why your oncologist may be talking about using additional therapy, even though your tumor has been removed by a surgeon or has been eliminated by chemotherapy and radiation. If the tumor is gone, why are we even talking about the relative benefit of continuing to undergo treatment? What is a relative benefit, anyway? Is this just some kind of insurance?

When I try to explain the benefits of adjuvant therapy, I draw stick figures on a piece of paper. Don't laugh. This is how relative benefit was explained to me when I was a fellow in oncology years ago, and I think it's the simplest way to understand why doctors so often recommend additional chemotherapy. Adjuvant chemotherapy should be offered only when it has been proven to improve the chance of cure in clinical trials.

These clinical trials have determined which adjuvant therapies are the best at eliminating those remaining cancer cells. In these trials, patients were placed at random into groups (arms). One group received surgery alone, and the other got surgery plus additional treatment such as chemotherapy or radiation—or both. At the end of five years, researchers looked at both groups to see how many had the cancer return. In the example given in figure 3.1, let's say that of the ten people with stage 3 colon cancer who had surgery alone, we know that six will be cured by surgery, while the remaining four will not. Those four will die from their cancer during the next five years. The trouble is that we don't know whether any one patient will be in the group that is cured or the group that will have the cancer return.

When we look at a similar group of ten patients who had surgery plus adjuvant chemotherapy, we see that seven of them have been cured by surgery plus chemotherapy, and the remaining three still

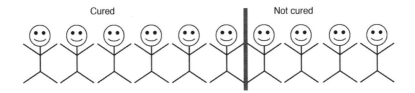

Cured   Not cured

Figure 3.1 Cured versus not cured without adjuvant chemotherapy

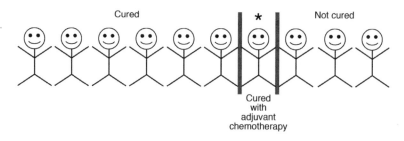

Figure 3.2 Cured versus not cured with surgery plus adjuvant chemotherapy

have their cancer return within five years (figure 3.2). How do we get that number? We know that patients with stage 3 colon cancer who receive adjuvant chemotherapy do 25 percent better relative to the group who had surgery alone. But that doesn't mean that the survival rate goes from 60 to 85 percent. Instead, it means that the death rate decreases by 25 percent. So, we have to multiply by 25 percent the number of patients who would otherwise not survive, which is four out of ten, or 40 percent. That gives us an absolute benefit for the entire group of ten at 10 percent. In figure 3.2, we can see that if all ten patients receive adjuvant chemotherapy, we can expect that seven out of ten will be cured, while the other three will see their cancer return even with chemotherapy.

What's frustrating is that six of those people would have been cured without adjuvant chemotherapy, and three were destined to have their cancer return even with adjuvant chemotherapy. Just one lucky person will be the beneficiary of all this extra therapy and have his or her cancer cells eliminated by it. This is why your doctor will talk to you about the possibility of having adjuvant chemotherapy.

You may benefit from having these chemotherapy treatments, but this all depends on your risk of dying from cancer over the next five years and the relative benefit of adjuvant chemotherapy for your type of cancer. These numbers vary for different types of cancers. Knowing these numbers and understanding what they mean will be important factors in your decision, because chemotherapy may mean months of additional treatments and side effects.

Next, I've outlined the statistics for patients with stage 3 colon cancer that has a very high likelihood of returning (figure 3.3). For

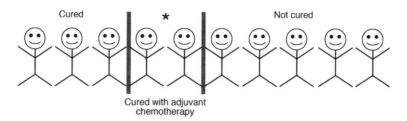

Figure 3.3   Benefit of adjuvant chemotherapy on less curable cancers

these patients, there is a 70 percent chance of dying from cancer during the next five years. For them, the absolute benefit of chemotherapy is 17.5 percent, a number we reach by multiplying 25 percent by 70 percent. This is a very different decision because you can opt for additional treatment that reduces the likelihood of dying in five years by almost 20 percent.

Lines of Treatment

When we describe a cancer as progressing, we mean that it is getting worse or failing to respond to treatment. A progressing cancer is continuing to divide, grow, and invade more tissues. You should also understand that cancer doesn't progress gradually from stage 1 to stage 2 and then 3. If you have been treated for stage 2 cancer and then it returns in a different location, it is always called metastatic or recurrent cancer. Even if you had stage 1 cancer initially, and then after several years we detect cancer in the liver, you are now metastatic. One of the confusing points of staging is that technically a cancer data registry is always supposed to record your stage as the stage you had when you first were diagnosed. But your cancer team will refer to you as having stage 4 cancer if any metastases are detected even if you first presented with stage 1 or 2 cancer.

With a stage 4 cancer, doctors often refer to a treatment as a line of therapy, because there are usually several standard treatments for each type of cancer. Researchers are always discovering and testing new therapies that are slightly more successful for a type of cancer. To keep all of these new therapies straight, several of the best academic centers in the country came together about twenty years ago to start the National Comprehensive Cancer Network. It is known among doctors as the NCCN. Oncologists from these centers gather yearly to determine the best treatments for each stage of cancer and to outline the best lines of therapy for each metastatic cancer. The guidelines produced by the NCCN help oncologists and patients (and insurance companies) to stay abreast of the best treatments. You might hear your oncologist talk about a treatment being "on the guidelines." He or she is usually talking about these NCCN guidelines.

Your doctor will start with what is known to be the most successful treatment for your type of cancer according to the NCCN guidelines, and that is known as the first-line treatment. If the cancer adapts to that treatment and grows through it, meaning that it continues to spread even after several rounds of chemotherapy, the doctor will switch to another treatment, and that will be called the second-line treatment.

We switch to another line of treatment when a cancer becomes resistant to the first treatment, meaning that the cells have figured out how to grow and divide despite chemotherapy being in your system. This may seem confusing, and you may be wondering why cancer is able to grow despite a chemotherapy that has worked well for many months or even years. But cancer medicine is the same as any other type of medicine. If you had an infection, such as a urinary tract infection, your doctor would try to eradicate it with an antibiotic, such as penicillin. Usually that works well, but if you have had chronic urinary tract infections, you would have been treated intermittently with penicillin until the bacteria in your body became resistant to it. Then, your doctor would switch you to another antibiotic, such as Bactrim or ciprofloxacin. And you would continue to use it until it became ineffective as well. Chemotherapy, which is just a term that means "chemical therapy," is really the same.

If your doctor has told you that your cancer is treatable but not curable, you should expect that at some point the cancer will grow through your current treatment and you will need to switch to a new regimen. Of course, we hope that is many months or years from now. Your oncologist is hoping for the same thing that you are hoping for, which is a long run on each regimen.

4

....

What Is a Liquid Tumor?

HEMATOLOGIC MALIGNANCIES ARE CANCERS OF the blood cells, and they include leukemia and lymphoma, myeloma, and bone marrow failure states. These cancers are so distinct from solid tumors that they deserve their own chapter. If you have any one of these so-called liquid tumors, you will have a different experience in diagnosis, staging, and prognosis than will patients who have solid tumors. Oncologists think very differently about these types of tumors and how to treat them.

The first difference is that hematologic cancers are often detected by routine blood tests. You may have been diagnosed before feeling any symptoms of a disorder, or, in the case of lymphoma, you may have experienced some swelling lymph nodes or night sweats. Subsequent blood tests and DNA tests will reveal whether the circulating abnormal cells are actually cancerous. More important, they can help determine what type of cancer they are.

These types of cancers don't always fall neatly into a single category, although any of them can ultimately lead to bone marrow failure. While an oncologist can usually classify a cancer as one of the four major types, the variability within each group is enormous. One patient's large-cell lymphoma is not the same as that of another patient with the same diagnosis.

Every year researchers publish new studies based on molecular pathology, which is the study of the genetic mutations in the cancer cell. This research continues to suggest new classifications and groupings of hematologic malignancies, along with new ways of approaching and treating these cancers. So the pace of change is dizzying. Because of these new developments, it's getting harder to treat these cancers without the help of a major academic center. If you live in a region with one of these large teaching hospitals, you may want to have your test results reviewed there.

The initial diagnosis and staging of one of these cancers requires special blood tests and bone marrow biopsies. We rely far less on scans for these malignancies, except in the case of lymphoma, where we do rely on scans to see the tumors and how the treatment is working.

Questions to Ask Your Oncologist

When friends contact me to say that a family member of theirs has received this kind of diagnosis, I tell them to ask the following questions of the oncologist:

- Is my type of cancer curable or incurable?
- Is my cancer aggressive or slow growing?
- Will I need to start treatment right away to get the best chance at a cure?
- Will I need aggressive treatments that might require a bone marrow transplant to get the best chance at a cure?

It may seem odd to have to ask the oncologist whether your cancer is curable, but you may have gone through lots of testing to get at a diagnosis, and patients and doctors alike sometimes skirt this issue. With solid tumors, the staging helps to determine whether a cancer is curable. We know that a stage 4 solid tumor is probably not. Most oncologists who specialize in hematologic cancers believe that many cancers, regardless of the stage, are potentially curable, even if the ultimate chance at a cure is lower than 50 percent. This changes the relationship between doctor and patient. The question you want to ask is *how* curable it is. In many of these cancers, age is a factor. A patient in her twenties might have an excellent chance for a cure. For example, Neal is a thirty-one-year-old who came to the clinic because of fevers and fatigue. A chest X-ray showed a mass in the middle of his chest, and then a PET-CT (see chapter 6 on the various types of scans and imaging used in cancer treatment) revealed multiple enlarged lymph nodes throughout his body. He now has a diagnosis of stage 4 Hodgkin's, a lymphoma of the white blood cells. Yet, despite the widespread nature of his cancer, Neal is likely to be cured with chemotherapy.

You also want to know how aggressive the cancer seems to be. If you have an aggressive hematologic malignancy, your doctor will want to start treatment immediately, and you may have already experienced a medical emergency that triggered your diagnosis. You won't have a lot of time to think about how much treatment and medical intervention you want to have at first. You still want to ask how much chemotherapy you will have to have to get a chance at a cure and whether the oncologist thinks that you might require a bone marrow transplant.

In contrast, if the cancer is indolent, meaning slow growing, you have time to get used to the diagnosis and to consider treatment options. Even if an indolent cancer is treatable but not curable, you will have years—perhaps many years—in which you work with your oncologist to keep the cancer in check, to manage its symptoms and side effects, and to live your life with this diagnosis.

Regardless of whether you are curable or incurable and regardless of your type of cancer, you will want to ask when treatment should begin to give you the best chance at a best-case scenario. Does it need to start immediately, or do you have a few weeks to get used to the diagnosis? And how disruptive is the treatment likely to be? How many weeks or months will it last? As a patient, you want to have an idea of what the future will look like for you. How many hospitalizations, how many side effects are likely if you decide to accept every treatment with the hope for a cure or to live as long as possible.

By asking this series of questions, you will get an excellent idea of the prognosis (the likely course and outcome of your disease) and treatment. You will also be able to come to terms with what is required for the best chance at the best-case scenario and how much treatment is right for you.

How Curable Is Leukemia?

These cancers are malignancies among the bone marrow cells, generally immature white blood cells. When these cells are overproduced, they crowd out functioning bone marrow cells and lead to anemia and other problems. You may have been told that you have one of the two types of leukemia, chronic or acute.

The chronic leukemias consist of chronic myelogenous leukemia (CML) and chronic lymphocytic leukemia (CLL). Chronic leukemias tend to be very treatable even if they aren't curable. Twenty years ago when I first started in oncology, CML was fatal unless you received a bone marrow transplant. And even then the cure rate was barely above 50 percent. But now CML is a chronic illness controlled for years on end by a pill. It's a dramatic success story. The survival rate for people with CML is almost as good as the survival rate for people without CML. CLL, however, can be an indolent disease until it starts to cause problems, and then patients require multiple chemotherapy regimens to keep it under control.

The acute leukemias are completely different. Acute myelogenous leukemia (AML) and acute lymphocytic leukemia (ALL) are medical emergencies when diagnosed. Patients are often admitted to the hospital right away and started on aggressive chemotherapy. Many patients with AML and ALL will require a bone marrow transplant to have the best chance at being cured. The road with AML and ALL can be a long one with multiple stays in the hospital.

I treated Josephine five years ago when she had a localized colon cancer. Thankfully, it was stage 1, and she didn't need any chemotherapy or radiation after her surgery. I continued to follow her for the next five years to make sure that the cancer didn't return, a period of care we call surveillance. At the end of that time, Josephine called me to say that she was extremely tired and she worried that the cancer had come back. She came in the next day and had blood drawn. During our clinical visit, her blood work popped up on my computer screen to show a white blood cell count of 115,000, a level ten times the normal range, and it was almost all blasts, or immature white blood cells. I knew immediately that she had AML. Josephine was admitted directly to the hospital to prepare for a regimen of chemotherapy to eliminate these AML blast cells, and she remained in the hospital for most of the next month. Unfortunately, the genetics of her AML showed that she had an extremely aggressive form and would need a bone marrow transplant if she wanted to be cured. The next two years are going to be hard for Josephine, as she will be in and out of the hospital for treatment.

As you can imagine, age and general health are both key factors in how aggressively your doctor can treat acute leukemias. The underlying genetics of leukemia also makes a huge difference in prognosis and treatment. Some mutations in the DNA carry a very poor prognosis, and patients with these mutations will require a bone marrow transplant for any reasonable chance at cure. Other mutations carry a very good prognosis with chemotherapy alone. Additionally, patients over the age of sixty can struggle to manage the side effects of aggressive chemotherapy. In general, patients over the age of seventy aren't offered bone marrow transplants, which are considered too dangerous at this age. The curability of acute leukemia declines as you get older.

How Curable Is Lymphoma?

Lymphomas are collections of cancerous blood cells growing in the lymph system. Indolent lymphomas are rarely curable, but patients can do extremely well with treatment because the cells aren't reproducing quickly and because they often respond well to treatment. Sometimes you can have a lymphoma and not need any treatment right away. If your lymphoma is indolent, you can expect to have a close relationship with your oncologist for years as you both monitor the disease and the intermittent treatment required.

The aggressive lymphomas are often more curable, but the treatments are aggressive and can involve a bone marrow transplant. If you're diagnosed with an aggressive lymphoma, you won't have weeks to decide what you want to do. Often your doctor will want to know your preferences that week because you're either very sick at that point or you will be shortly. If you have an aggressive lymphoma and it's potentially curable, as they often are, then you'll need to decide quickly whether you want to go down the path to cure.

How Curable Is Myeloma?

Unfortunately, myeloma is very rarely curable. Nevertheless, new treatments in the past ten years have made the prognosis for patients with myeloma much better. Patients with myeloma can often live productive lives for five years or more before they get sick from their cancer. Myeloma is different from the other hematologic malignancies in that the tumors secrete proteins called immunoglobulins that we can measure and follow during the course of treatment. These proteins can also cause damage to other organs, particularly the kidneys. Dealing with the side effects of these proteins and kidney damage can be a major focus of both the treatment and the supportive care that patients receive.

How Curable Is Myelodysplastic Syndrome?

This is a group of bone marrow disorders that cause bone marrow failure. The disorder is exactly what it seems to be. Your bone marrow can't make enough red cells, white cells, and platelets to keep you alive. Unfortunately, myelodysplastic syndrome (MDS) isn't curable without a bone marrow transplant. Even with a transplant, MDS is not often cured. It usually occurs in older adults who are not candidates for bone marrow transplant. In this case, your doctor will work with you to relieve your symptoms and slow down the failure of the bone marrow, if possible.

Staging

Hematologic malignancies are staged differently than solid tumors are, and the traditional TNM stage of cancer is less predictive of your chance at a cure; indeed, it may be irrelevant. You may know someone with a solid tumor, and if so, you know that staging relies on the size of the tumor in the organ where it started along with how far it has spread in the body. If a solid tumor has spread to the lymph nodes or to another organ, you know that the cancer is at an advanced stage. In solid tumors, oncologists use biopsies, scans, and other tests to determine staging.

In hematologic malignancies, doctors use blood tests as a starting point to identify abnormal cells. But, once there is a suspicion of cancer, your doctor knows that he or she has to look at the source of those abnormal cells, meaning the bone marrow, to see how many abnormal cells there are and how aggressive they are.

Bone marrow is the spongy center of your largest bones, and it contains the stem cells that create all the blood cells in your body. These cells are created in the bone marrow and then mature over the course of a few days. In your bone marrow at any one time, there are red blood cells and white blood cells and platelets in various stages of maturation. In the case of leukemia, the bone marrow will contain an unusual number of cells that are stuck at an immature phase of development and yet are multiplying. In the case of acute leukemia, such as AML or ALL, these cells are stuck at the earliest stage of development, called a blast, and have filled up the bone marrow and have even spilled out into the bloodstream. Chronic leukemias, such as CML or CLL, will show more mature cells that look more like normal white blood cells. But there will simply be too many of them. Over several years, they will squeeze out production of other types of blood cells and cause problems.

None of this information about what's going on inside the bone marrow is available through simple blood tests. So your doctor will probably order a bone marrow biopsy. It sounds intimidating, but the procedure is actually completely routine.

The Bone Marrow Biopsy

Most of your bone marrow is located in three areas: the sternum, vertebrae, and pelvis. The easiest and safest way to get a sample of bone marrow is with a needle biopsy into the pelvis.

For a bone marrow biopsy, you will be asked to change into a hospital gown and then lie on your stomach on an exam table. The usual spot for a biopsy of this kind is an area on your back called the iliac crest. If you feel the top of your hip bone on your side and then follow the top of that bone to your back just below the area of your kidneys, you'll find the spot where the needle will go in. Don't worry about that part yet. First the area will be cleaned with iodine. Then the doctor or nurse will inject lidocaine, a pain medication, to numb both the skin and the bone marrow. If you are especially nervous, you can take pain medication or antianxiety medication as well about fifteen minutes before the procedure.

By the time the needle biopsy itself has started, you will feel pressure as the needle enters the iliac crest. The doctor will take two samples of bone marrow. First, he or she will draw back on the syringe and remove some of the liquid bone marrow. This is often the most painful part of the biopsy. The sudden draw of the syringe can cause a brief, sharp pain in the hip. The second part of the biopsy is a core biopsy, in which the doctor will take about a one-centimeter piece of bone marrow. This will feel like someone is pushing down hard on your hip. It shouldn't hurt, but you will feel the pressure. And then you're done. You will be able to get up and go home. After the lidocaine wears off, you will be sore for a couple of days. You may have a bruise, but there is often no visible sign that you've had a procedure at all, except for the Band-Aid that was put over the site.

In the lab, both the liquid and solid components are prepared so that we can look at them under the microscope. We can often tell by how the cells look (i.e., its morphology) what type of cancer you have and how extensive it is. But we almost never rely on morphology today. The DNA tests on the bone marrow often tell the story of exactly what type of cancer you have and what the treatment and prognosis are. These tests will take several days to even a few weeks to come back.

Ultimately, the bone marrow biopsy is giving your medical team a more complete picture of your hematologic malignancy. Sometimes, the blood tests can tell your doctor most of what's needed to confirm the diagnosis. In this case, the bone marrow biopsy is a final confirmation of both the stage and type of cancer cells that are causing the problem. In other cases, such as leukemia and bone marrow failure, the biopsy gives critical information about the state of your bone marrow and what the cancer cells in it are up to.

Scans in Lymphoma

The third major staging need for hematologic cancers is imaging, which is primarily done for lymphomas to see whether the lymph nodes throughout the body are involved and whether the cancer is invading the organs.

Even in solid tumors, the lymph nodes are a significant part of staging. Your lymph system runs throughout your body and follows the venous system. Lymph is milky liquid that circulates through your body and contains white blood cells, specifically the B and T cells that fight both infection and cancer. The lymph nodes are larger pockets containing these cells. When you are fighting an illness, they tend to become swollen as they work to isolate and destroy invading bacteria. They also swell when they are invaded by cancer cells. A normal lymph node is less than one centimeter in size, and usually less than five millimeters. A lymph node that has swollen to a size larger than one centimeter may contain cancer cells. Your doctor may order a PET scan as a way to look at the lymph nodes and see what's going on. In fact, a PET scan is so valuable in seeing cancer cells in the lymph system that patients will often have several of these scans over time to see how the lymphoma is responding to treatment.

Looking at the Brain

The last step of staging is to look at the brain. Hematologic cancers can often hide out in the brain, where standard chemotherapies can't reach them. There is a blood-brain barrier that separates the circulating blood from the cerebrospinal fluid in the nervous system. Your doctor will want to look at the cerebrospinal fluid, located in the brain or spinal cord, to see whether any of these white or red blood cells are circulating in it. If so, the cancer may have migrated to this fluid.

Your doctor may order a magnetic resonance imaging (MRI) of the brain and then order a spinal tap to sample the spinal fluid to check it for these red or white blood cells. Again, this may sound like a difficult procedure, but is fairly simple.

The Spinal Tap

In this procedure, you will lie on your side while the doctor inserts a small needle in the space between two vertebrae in your lower back. If you've had an epidural while giving birth, this will feel exactly the same. The doctor will numb the area beforehand and then use a needle to remove a few milliliters of cerebrospinal fluid. The procedure should be relatively painless. Afterward, you may have a headache, called a spinal headache, because of the changes to the levels of spinal fluid circulating in your central nervous system. You can take acetaminophen and fluids to treat it, but it should last just a day or two. In rare instances, the needle can cause a small tear in the compartment that holds the spinal fluid in place, and in that case you might require a blood patch. For this, a doctor will inject a small amount of your blood directly into the area of the first injection so that it can repair the tear. Thankfully, this is an unusual complication.

Parameters of Staging

After we have the peripheral blood, the bone marrow, the scans (CT, PET, and MRI), and the brain evaluated, we have completed the staging of your hematologic cancer. At this point, it's important to ask whether there is any confusion in the diagnosis. For most hematologic malignancies, there is little confusion. The leukemias and myelomas are usually straightforward diagnoses. One source of confusion in the diagnosis of leukemias may be that the genetics are inconclusive. The genetics of leukemias often determine the likelihood of success and cure with a particular treatment. Sometimes the genetics of a particular leukemia aren't straightforward, and there may be disagreement among experts on the best way to approach treatment.

While most lymphomas are straightforward pathologic diagnoses, different subtypes of lymphomas are being recognized all the time, and these distinctions can have a profound impact on treatment. A pathologic diagnosis of lymphoma can be very difficult, and if you are at a community hospital or cancer center, it may be beneficial to ask that the pathology slides be read by a lymphoma expert in pathology at the closest academic medical center.

The staging of hematologic cancers does give us an idea of the curability of a certain cancer. So your oncologist should tell you which stage of cancer you have. And, as is the case with solid tumors, the stages are classed with the numbers 1 through 4. Still, your stage 4 lymphoma is not like your aunt's stage 4 breast cancer. Stage 4 large-cell lymphoma is often quite curable while stage 4 solid tumors are rarely curable. Most hematologic cancers have prognostic scoring systems associated with them, and you should ask your oncologist how your tumor scored on these systems.

Hematologic malignancy experts look at staging and these scoring systems as a way to tell us how much tumor burden someone has, meaning roughly how many cancer cells are being produced. The higher the tumor burden, the less curable the cancer and the more side effects someone is likely to suffer from treatment. The lower the tumor burden, the more curable the cancer and the less likely someone is to suffer side effects.

Choosing Treatment Options

With hematologic malignancies there is often a chance of curing people who have advanced cancer by using very aggressive therapy. In solid tumors, we know quickly after staging whether someone has a chance at a cure or not. As a result, oncologists who specialize in these liquid tumors are always looking for a way to try to cure you, even if that means using extremely aggressive chemotherapy that will require a bone marrow transplant. Of course, as you get older, there is a greater likelihood that these aggressive treatments can be difficult, and you may have to consider how your body will tolerate them.

In the beginning, you may be convinced that you will endure anything to have a chance at a cure, and that's great, but over the course of treatment, your feelings may change, and you want to be able to communicate these feelings to your medical team. You want to work with an oncologist who understands you and your goals for treatment, someone who is a good communicator and a good listener.

Bone Marrow Transplant

Many hematologic malignancies can be cured—even if they are widespread—by a bone marrow transplant. This is the process of replacing damaged stem cells in the bone marrow with healthy cells. These healthy cells can come from your own body or from a donor (see chapter 14). These new stem cells can then create a new generation of white blood cells that can attack the cancer cells in your bone marrow and blood stream. When it is effective, this is called the graft versus leukemia (or lymphoma) effect.

As miraculous as a successful bone marrow transplant can be, it also carries serious risks. If the grafted stem cells were taken from your own body, they will likely take hold without many complications. But if they come from a donor, which is called an allogeneic transplant, they can cause problems. The new white blood cells that come from a donor may be incompatible at first with your system. In this case, these new white cells can view your normal cells as foreign and attack them. This is called graft versus host disease. Allogeneic bone marrow transplants were extremely dangerous when they were first introduced in 1958. At that time, the mortality from the procedure was roughly 30 percent, which means that nearly one-third of all people who had them died of complications from the procedure. Another 30 percent of people were completely cured of their cancer. These numbers have improved over the years, but you should definitely talk to your doctor about the risks of developing life-threatening complications from a transplant. It is also critical that you get your physical symptoms aggressively treated while you are going through a bone marrow transplant. New data from our institution shows that patients who are undergoing this procedure who have a palliative care consultation during transplant have a much better quality of life and lower rates of depression and anxiety.

When to Start Treatment

Your oncologist should be able to tell you whether your cancer is indolent or aggressive. An indolent cancer has probably been in your system for many months or years prior to your diagnosis. You have time to digest the diagnosis and make a decision about when to start treatment. This is again different from solid tumors, in which doctors usually want to start treatment right away to have the best chance at a best-case scenario.

If your cancer is aggressive, your doctor will warn you that you can get sick very quickly. In fact, you may have been admitted to the hospital at the time of diagnosis because of a medical emergency related to the cancer. In that case, you will have to make decisions within the first few days about starting treatment. This can feel overwhelming. If you have a chance at a cure, this will influence your decision. But if you have no chance at a cure, or if you are elderly, you may want to think about how much medical intervention you want and how difficult it will be to endure before you make a decision. It's important not to be isolated while thinking about these things. Spouses and immediate family members can help you think about what you value and what you really want from your medical team. If you have no spouse or immediate family, a trusted friend can help you navigate these decisions.

Also, give your doctor permission to talk about what he or she would do in your situation and why. If your doctor is younger than you are, ask what she would do if you were her mom or dad. If your doctor is much older, ask what he would do if you were his child. This is your first time in this situation, but your oncologist has talked to and helped hundreds of people in this situation and is probably expecting these questions from you.

Unfortunately, some doctors are uncomfortable with these questions and refuse to answer them. I welcome these questions because they allow me to talk to patients about their goals and values.

5

How to Prepare for Treatment

STARTING TREATMENT CAN BE UNNERVING because you don't know what to expect and because this is the part where you become a patient being treated for cancer. You may have had surgery already and everything may feel very surreal. This time is one of the toughest because you don't know how your body is going to respond to treatment. You don't yet know how to trust this new body, but you will. You will become a competent, capable cancer patient. I wish you didn't have to, but you will.

In this chapter, I'm going to talk you through everything you need to know to prepare for radiation or chemotherapy. First, I'll explain the basics of radiation therapy and how to prepare for it. Then, I'll explain what chemotherapy is and how different classes of chemotherapy work. I'll describe a typical day in the infusion unit, the facility inside the hospital or clinic where chemotherapy is provided. I'll also tell you what you need to know about side effects, and how you can adjust your schedule for chemotherapy to better fit into your life.

What Is Radiation Therapy?

This is one of the mainstays of cancer treatment, because radiation kills cancer cells by damaging their DNA. If the cells have enough radiation damage, then they will die when they go to divide. Many cancer cells don't divide for four to eight weeks, which is why it often takes two months to see the optimum effect of radiation therapy.

People sometimes ask why we can't apply radiation therapy to the whole body if it works this well to kill cancer cells. The answer is that radiation damages normal tissues in the same way that it damages cancer cells. So doctors think of radiation as a local therapy that should be directed at tumors alone. You can think of it the same way you would think about surgery, except without the incision and the pain.

There are two types of radiation therapy: internal and external. For internal radiation therapy—also called brachytherapy—a radiation oncologist places radioactive beads inside the body next to a tumor. Brachytherapy is sometimes used for patients with local tumors in the prostate, breast, and cervix, but there are limited applications for this kind of therapy. The most common form of radiation therapy is external beam radiation. A machine called a linear accelerator produces a beam of radiation therapy that goes into and through your body.

Why Do I Need Radiation?

There are several reasons doctors recommend radiation instead of surgery or in addition to chemotherapy. Some people are not good candidates for surgery, while others have a type of tumor that might be equally treatable with radiation or surgery. For example, men with prostate cancer often debate the merits of surgical removal of the tumor versus primary radiation therapy to treat a localized prostate tumor. Sometimes elderly patients with lung cancer are treated with primary radiation therapy because thoracic surgery to remove a lung cancer is deemed too dangerous.

Doctors also recommend radiation therapy in addition to surgery when there is a strong suspicion that microscopic cancer cells may remain around the site after the tumor has been removed. This is called adjuvant radiation therapy. Even if a surgeon has cut a wide swath around the tumor, patients can still be at risk of another tumor developing from those cells that were left behind. If the tumor was large or if there were a number of lymph nodes that showed metastases, that is, the spread of cancer cells to another location, doctors may suspect that there are cancer cells in the tissues surrounding the tumor that weren't removed. Some cancers are like jellyfish in that they grow tentacles outward from the central tumor and these can't be seen on scans. If there is a high chance that some cells remain after surgery, your doctor may want to use radiation on that area to have a better chance of killing those cells. If you get radiation prior to surgery to help shrink the tumor, this is called neoadjuvant radiation therapy. Adjuvant and neoadjuvant radiation should be used only when evidence from clinical trials supports it.

Radiation can also be used to reduce symptoms from metastatic cancer. In fact, it's a wonderful way to reduce or even eliminate pain from metastatic sites, including bone metastases. It can also stop cancers from bleeding or growing into vital structures such as the spinal cord.

The Planning Session

Everyone who gets radiation therapy undergoes a planning session, often called a simulation, or "sim." This planning session can often take an hour to complete. The radiation oncologist and radiation physicist will position your body so that multiple beams of radiation will cross the area of the tumor. By using multiple beams of radiation, the radiation oncologist can concentrate the highest dose around the cancer and limit the amount of radiation therapy normal tissues see.

When they have figured out the appropriate position for your body, one of them will place a small tattoo on the skin as a reference point. This ensures that the radiation therapist can position you correctly for each session of radiation. The tattoo is usually a small blue dot the size of a pen mark. Correct positioning is critical, and that's why you will receive a small tattoo. If you have tumors in the brain, head, and neck, you might need to be fitted with a mask that will be used with each radiation treatment to make sure that the beam is in exactly the right position.

The radiation oncology team will discuss all of this with you and take you through it step by step. It can sound daunting, but just like with chemotherapy, once you learn the ropes and your team, it will all feel easier.

How Much Radiation Will I Need?

You may be scheduled to receive either a long course or a short course of radiation. In a long course, smaller amounts of radiation are delivered every day over an extended time, perhaps four to six weeks. In short course radiation therapy, larger doses of radiation are delivered every day over an abbreviated period, such as one week. There are pros and cons to the different schedules of radiation for each tumor type.

The dose of radiation that any patient receives is measured in Grays, named after Henry Louis Gray, one of the pioneers in X-ray technology. A Gray is often abbreviated Gy. Each Gy is equivalent to one joule of energy absorbed per kilogram of tissue. The total amount of Gys that are required to kill a tumor is dependent on the individual tumor, but many tumors require 40 to 70 Gy to be killed. By comparison, a CT scan has 16 mGy, or 0.16 Gy. The amount of radiation delivered with each dose is called a fraction, and this is also measured in Gy.

You will typically need to arrive for radiation at the same time each day, and you will usually have the same radiation therapist to position you on the table and direct the radiation based on the location of your small tattoo. The radiation itself will be over in just a few minutes, but the entire visit to the radiation oncology department will generally take thirty to forty-five minutes. Like everything else, you will get used to the routine, and the staff will be able to get you in and out pretty quickly. I have had many patients tell me that they become friendly with the other patients getting radiation at the same time because you do see each other every day for up to several weeks. You become radiation buddies. When you complete a course of radiation at MGH, you get to ring a bell in the waiting room if you want. It becomes a celebratory moment to mark completion of the course.

Side Effects of Radiation

There are both short- and long-term side effects to radiation.

Fatigue. This is the most common immediate side effect of radiation. I tell my patients to expect to be exhausted beginning about two weeks after the radiation starts and lasting until two weeks after it ends. People who never needed an afternoon nap before will find themselves napping regularly. This will subside over the course of about a month, but I encourage people to think about how they will manage this fatigue so they are prepared.

Inflammation. Although the treatment itself is painless, radiation does cause some short-term swelling in soft tissues. This swelling can cause pain, but it is generally temporary. The specific side effects you may experience will depend on the location of the tumor and the direction of the radiation. If a tumor is close to the skin, you may develop what looks like a sunburn in that area. If radiation hits the gastrointestinal tract, you may develop nausea or diarrhea.

Scarring. The normal tissues in the path of radiation beams can sustain long-term damage. For women who receive radiation to the underarm for breast cancer, this scarring can cause the affected arm to swell. If radiation has hit the digestive tract, you can get scarring that causes obstructions there. Occasionally, vital organs can be scarred, including the heart and kidneys, and this can lead to long-term damage. Radiation oncologists do everything they can to avoid vital organs, but sometimes the location of the tumor doesn't allow for this.

Bone marrow suppression. Radiation can damage the stem cells in your bone marrow, which can impair the production of blood cells in your body. You may have low blood counts after getting radiation to certain parts of your bone marrow. Usually, your body can bounce back quickly.

Pneumonitis. Sometimes patients can develop pneumonitis, or inflammation of the lung, if a portion of a lung has been radiated. This can sometimes be serious, and if you experience a cough or shortness of breath, you should call your oncologist. These symptoms can occur several weeks after the radiation is done. Sometimes we need to treat pneumonitis with steroids.

Cancer. The risk of developing a new radiation-induced cancer in the area that was radiated is about 1 percent over the course of the next twenty years. Still, this is a serious consideration that must be weighed against the beneficial effects of radiation for treating cancer. Tissues at high risk of developing cancer are those in young people that are still growing. That's why doctors do everything they can to limit the amount of radiation to hit normal tissues in children and adolescents.

What Is Proton Beam Radiation?

Conventional radiation uses photons or X-rays that enter and exit the body. With protons, by contrast, there is no exit dose of radiation beyond the tumor. Instead, a narrow concentration of radiation is delivered to the tumor itself. In essence, radiation oncologists can "paint" the radiation around the tumor more precisely and limit the normal tissues receiving radiation.

Proton beam therapy is not more effective at killing the cancer. It's merely more effective at limiting the long-term side effects of radiation. In some tumors, such as brain tumors in children, the advantages are obvious. But the advantages are less obvious in most adult solid tumors, and studies are under way comparing photons to protons. Generally, proton beam therapy is not considered standard care, and we do not offer it to solid tumor patients unless they are enrolled in a clinical trial.

What Is Chemotherapy?

Chemotherapy in its broadest sense is chemical therapy. Really, all of medicine is the use of chemicals to treat people. But, chemotherapy has come to mean any anticancer medication. Chemotherapy can be subdivided into four major categories: traditional cytotoxic chemotherapy, hormonal therapy, immunotherapy, and targeted therapy. Each of these categories carries different side effects that can be easy or difficult to tolerate, and each can be administered in several ways. They can be given intravenously (through the vein), orally (by mouth), or subcutaneously (under the skin).

Traditional cytotoxic chemotherapy kills cancer cells usually by damaging their DNA in some way. This is the category of chemotherapy with which most people are familiar. It can cause nausea, hair loss, low blood counts, and all the other traditional side effects associated with chemotherapy. It can be given by an intravenous infusion or orally. Just because a drug can be given orally doesn't necessarily mean that it's better tolerated or safer for the patient.

Hormonal therapy kills cancer cells that are dependent on being fed by hormones in your body, specifically estrogen and testosterone. Many breast cancers respond remarkably well to antiestrogens. The side effects are often quite manageable when compared with traditional cytotoxic chemotherapy, but these treatments can cause problems such as early menopause, osteoporosis, cataracts, and other long-term complications caused by low estrogen. In much the same way, prostate cancer feeds off testosterone. Prostate cancers will stop in their tracks and often die as soon as you remove testosterone from the system. We can do this by surgically removing the testicles or by administering antitestosterone medications. Removing testosterone, however, can produce many long-term side effects such as diminished energy level, weight gain, increased risks of heart attacks, osteoporosis, diminished libido, and erectile dysfunction.

Of course, these side effects can be very disruptive. Sometimes patients feel that their oncologists don't pay enough attention to their complaints about these deeply personal bodily changes. Oncologists can sometimes seem to dismiss these upheavals because they have patients dealing with life-threatening side effects from other therapies. I hope this isn't the case for you, because your oncologist should be taking these side effects seriously. One of the major contributions we have made as palliative care clinicians is to help the oncologists recognize the impact hormonal agents can have on the overall well-being of patients.

Immunotherapy treatments are chemicals or proteins that are designed to augment or activate immune cells to fight the cancer.

Typically, these regimens have none of the usual side effects associated with traditional cytotoxic chemotherapy that you receive in the infusion unit. So we often won't use antinausea medicines, and we are not worried about hair loss or low blood counts. But they can activate the immune system to such a degree that it can accidentally start attacking normal tissues and organs.

For instance, Jim is a fifty-eight-year-old man with melanoma who was prescribed immunotherapy. Every three weeks he was scheduled to come to the infusion unit for a one-hour visit in which the nurse would give him the drug intravenously. He felt fine at the time of his first infusion and for the next couple of days, but during the second week after receiving the drug, he started to have severe diarrhea, occasionally as often as seven or eight times per day. Other than the diarrhea, he felt fine. It turns out that the immunotherapy that Jim was receiving was causing his T cells—immune cells—to attack his colon. When he had a colonoscopy, it looked just like ulcerative colitis, an autoimmune disease where a patient's immune cells attack his or her colon. In fact, many of the new immunotherapy medications are causing autoimmune diseases as their main form of toxicity. Thankfully, most go away when you stop the medication.

Targeted therapy refers to medications that target a specific protein pathway that the cancer cells are using to survive. For this type of treatment, we rely on the molecular pathologist to study the DNA of the cancer cell and tell us whether a mutation that the tumor has is creating too much or too little of a specific protein, which may be allowing the cells to grow out of control. For certain mutations, there are treatments that shut down the protein pathway and allow the cells to die naturally. In chapter 2, Dave describes the importance of determining the genetic defects of the cancer, and targeted therapy is directed at these defects.

These medications can be given intravenously, usually when they are antibodies against a specific protein, or orally, often called targeted therapies. Your oncologist may refer to them as tyrosine kinase inhibitors. These tyrosine kinase inhibitors have very different kinds of side effects compared with standard chemotherapy. You probably won't experience nausea or low blood counts. But you may experience reactions such as rashes and sometimes specific organ toxicities. For instance, Sarah is a forty-nine-year-old woman who is receiving a targeted therapy against a protein called HER2 for her breast cancer. After about six months on the therapy, she started to get short of breath when she was climbing the stairs. It turns out that the medication was affecting her heart muscle. When her oncologist stopped the drug, her heart muscle returned to normal, and she could walk without a problem. There are times when a targeted therapy is doing a great job of controlling the cancer, and yet it causes such severe side effects that it needs to be stopped.

Targeted therapies have been one of the major advances in the past ten years of oncology, and their use has dramatically enhanced our understanding of how cancers become resistant to different medications. If you are fortunate to have the type of cancer that responds to a targeted therapy, you should know that the cancer will likely become resistant to this treatment at some point. It's similar to the way in which chronic infections eventually become resistant to a certain antibiotic. Oncologists are now using repeat biopsies of cancer cells that have become resistant to a targeted treatment to see whether another targeted therapy will be effective.

Sometimes, oncologists use a combination of several types of drugs to treat cancer. It can often get confusing for patients and their families, but asking about which class of drugs your treatment falls into will help you keep track of the kinds of side effects you can expect. It will also help you better understand what your team is trying to accomplish.

Getting Ready for Chemotherapy

There are several questions you will want to ask your doctor about chemotherapy to help you get oriented before you start. Even if you have already started treatment, these questions will spark important conversations about treatment and how you can better prepare yourself:

- What is a cycle of chemotherapy?
- How many cycles will I need before we will know how well the treatment is working?

- How long are the infusions? What will that day entail?
- What medications do I need to take before the infusion, or what medications will be given during the infusion?
- What are the common side effects for this regimen?
- What medications will I need to take to cope with side effects?
- Who do I call if I have unexpected side effects or if I need something?
- What about my fertility? (Of course, this isn't applicable for every patient.)

What Is a Cycle of Chemotherapy?

Chemotherapy is like many medical treatments in that you will need several of them to get good results, and a standard grouping of these treatments is called a cycle. Oncologists think solely in terms of cycles of chemotherapy. Every type of chemotherapy has a different measurement that constitutes a cycle. For regimens that are given weekly, a cycle usually refers to four weeks of treatment. For regimens that are given every other week or every three weeks, each treatment will usually be considered its own cycle. For oral regimens, oncologists usually label a cycle as a month of therapy, because most of these regimens have a set number of days that you will be taking the drug. Sometimes you get these medications continuously, and sometimes these medications are given for a set number of weeks followed by a set number of weeks off of the medication. These are rough guidelines, and you should always ask your oncologist what he or she considers a cycle for your specific chemotherapy regimen.

So your doctor should be able to tell you how many treatments you will need to complete a cycle and how many cycles of treatment you will need to complete before tests will show how well the treatment is working. Your doctor is also going to be monitoring how your body reacts to chemotherapy at different points in a cycle, so that he or she can adjust the dosage for the next cycle if you experience toxicity.

What Is Toxicity?

All chemotherapy regimens cause some side effects, but your doctor is going to be checking to see whether you are developing what's called toxicity. It sounds serious, but really it means any side effect caused by the medication.

Some toxicities are so mild that we hardly pay any attention to them. For instance, some drugs will cause mouth sores that last for a day or two. Other toxicities can be life threatening, and we have to follow you closely. Luckily, you don't have to worry about what these kinds of toxicities are because we are often following them by checking your labs. Certain toxicities can happen at the beginning, middle, or end of a cycle, and your doctor will be monitoring your health to check for them. If your doctor is concerned about toxicity affecting your health, he or she may decide to give you a lower dose of the chemotherapy during the next cycle. Some patients try to argue with oncologists who want to reduce the dosage. You should know that lowering the dose of chemotherapy won't necessarily reduce its efficacy. Instead, the oncologist is trying to make sure that your body can tolerate the treatment.

What Is an Infusion Like?

Intravenous chemotherapies are referred to as infusions. The length of the actual infusion will be different for each regimen of chemotherapy. Some are relatively short, an hour, and some can take up to eight hours, so it's good to ask how long the infusion will take for your type of chemotherapy. A few regimens require a two-day infusion, but that doesn't mean you will be in the hospital for two days. Instead, the infusion will be started via IV in the infusion unit, and then you will go home with a portable pump and come back two days later to have it disconnected.

While in the infusion unit, you will be attended to by nurses who are experts at answering your questions about the process and at making you more comfortable. They can get you blankets and ice chips and help keep you updated on the progress of the infusion. In some hospitals you will have the same infusion nurse throughout your treatment, and he or she will get to know you really well and will be an enormous asset during this time.

In addition to administering the actual infusion, these nurses are carrying out the important function of double-checking the doses of the medications that have been ordered and checking with the pharmacy to see when they will be mixed. Infusion nurses are also communicating with your doctor about how you are doing on any given day. If you are being given extra medications or fluids through your IV to help with side effects, infusion nurses know exactly what these are and why they are being given. So if you have questions about anything, this is the person to ask. Infusion nurses also have a lot of information and tips about how to deal with side effects.

Do I Need a Portacath?

We sometimes recommend that people who are getting intravenous chemotherapy get a portacath, also called a port. These are special venous access devices that are implanted under your skin (figure 5.1). The port is a disk with a chamber that attaches to an intravenous catheter, so that the infusions can be delivered into your bloodstream. This prevents the nurses from having to insert an IV line into your arm with every infusion, and it allows nurses to easily do a blood draw without searching for a vein in the arm. But it's not merely a convenience for infusion nurses. Many patients hate the constant sticks in the arm that it can take to find a vein for infusions. And after several months of infusions, some of the veins can become scarred and difficult to access.

An interventional radiologist or surgeon at your hospital can insert the port during a procedure that generally takes about forty-five minutes. You will receive local anesthesia to numb your skin along with intravenous medications to lessen any pain and anxiety. When the procedure is finished and the local anesthesia wears off, you will feel some discomfort that should resolve over the course of a day. It's fine to take acetaminophen or oxycodone for a day or two to ease the discomfort.

The port will look like a half-dollar just underneath the skin below your collarbone. An infusion nurse can insert a needle into the

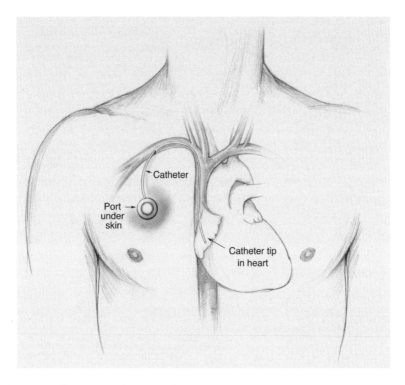

Figure 5.1 Placement of portacath

port to give you intravenous medications or fluids, or to take a blood draw (figure 5.2).

Some chemotherapy drugs can be given only through a port because they are too toxic to administer through smaller peripheral veins. If you are receiving one of these regimens, your only options are to have a port or to have a peripherally inserted central catheter (PICC) placed. PICCs are long IV catheters that you can leave in place for weeks at a time, but they are less convenient because you have to leave the IV taped to your arm for the entire time that you have it. By contrast, a port is covered entirely by your skin, so when it's not being accessed, you can swim and shower without damaging it.

There are two major concerns about ports, however. The first is that they can become infected, so anyone who accesses the port has to use sterile technique. Ports can also clot, and they can be a source

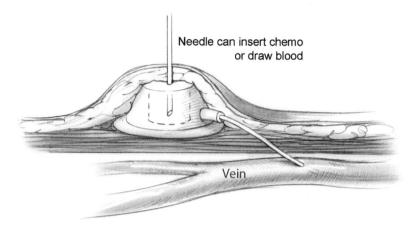

Needle can insert chemo or draw blood

Vein

Figure 5.2 Inserting a needle into portacath

of blood clots that can travel to the lung. If a port becomes infected or clotted, it almost always has to be removed. Ultimately, you should ask your doctor whether a port is right for you.

What Is a Day of Chemo Like?

While the infusion itself may take only a short time, a typical day in the clinic is likely to be much longer. Like most everything associated with medical treatment, there will be several necessary steps you have to go through along with some waiting around. To get an infusion, all these steps have to happen in order:

- A nurse or technician draws some blood so that the lab can do a complete blood count.
- You meet your clinician, either your oncologist or the nurse practitioner, for a checkup.
- The clinician checks your blood work and orders the chemotherapy to be mixed in the pharmacy.
- You go to the infusion unit and wait for a room or chair to be available.
- The nurse sets up your IV.
- The chemotherapy drugs are delivered to the floor and double-checked by your nurse.

- You get medications or fluids to prepare for chemotherapy.
- Your nurse administers the infusion.

Sometimes the lab gets backed up doing blood counts, sometimes your clinician is running late because of an emergency, and sometimes the pharmacy gets overwhelmed with chemotherapy orders. So the infusion may not start exactly at the appointed time. I had a patient, Stan, who was a grade school teacher, and very meticulous. During one of our first appointments, he stood to excuse himself, telling me that he had to hurry to the infusion unit because his appointment was at 10 a.m. exactly. I had to tell him that the nurses on the unit weren't expecting him exactly at his appointment time. They know that they can't give an infusion until the blood work comes in, the clinician orders the chemo, and the lab has mixed it. In this case, it's okay to just relax and go with the process.

I find that patients do best when they plan to spend an entire day in the infusion unit by bringing something to do, a book to read, movies to watch, or a loved one or friend to spend some of the day with them. Then, if things run really smoothly and they are done in a few hours, they consider it a bonus.

There are several things you can do to help speed things along:

- *Get the blood work done early.* If you arrive thirty to forty-five minutes before your appointment time to have the blood drawn, you will have a better chance of having the labs back when you see your clinician. Then you can get right to the infusion unit.
- *Keep a log of what you experience after each infusion.* The doctor is going to ask a lot of predictable questions about your bowels, how much you ate, whether you were in any pain, how long you were fatigued. Having ready answers means that the doctor has the best information and can make decisions based on how your body is reacting to treatment.
- *Have your list of questions ready for your clinician.* Your doctor will be asking you about side effects and the doses of medications you are taking to control side effects. If you have a list of questions or concerns about side effects or can detail how you felt after the previous infusion, your doctor can help you with those

right away, and you won't worry that you are forgetting something. If you have questions about when you will be getting scans or how your blood work looks, this is the time to ask.

Additional Medications

After you get to the infusion unit and your nurse has the chemotherapy mixed for you in hand, you will get different medications to help with the side effects of the chemotherapy. You might get anti-nausea medications like ondansetron, which are more fully explained in chapter 9. These drugs dramatically reduce the nausea that patients experience from chemotherapy. You might have been instructed to take some steroids the night before the chemotherapy infusion. Taking all these medications as prescribed is crucial to minimize the side effects of the chemotherapy infusion.

Allergic Reactions

Many people have allergies of some kind, and most people know of someone who is allergic to some class of medication. Chemotherapy is no different in that there are some people who have, or develop, an allergic reaction to the chemotherapy drug they are being given. Rest assured that infusion nurses are experts in seeing and treating even mild allergic reactions. This is one of the reasons they will be constantly checking on you to see how you are responding to each infusion.

Most times an allergic reaction is mild, such as a single hive on your arm. It's rare but possible for certain patients to develop an overwhelming allergic reaction, called anaphylaxis, in which the tongue will begin to tingle and swell and they may start to wheeze or cough. In some people a reaction is preceded by a funny feeling in the head or body, and, in a few of these cases, people have a severe and sudden reaction in which they pass out before they know what's happening. Know that a capable nurse will be steps away from you at all times during your infusion and that if you do have even a mild reaction, your nurse will stop your infusion immediately and give you medications such as steroids and antihistamines to stop it.

Patients who do have a severe reaction may have to see an allergist to undergo desensitization to the chemotherapy, just as you would undergo desensitization to penicillin if you were allergic and really needed it.

Side Effects

You probably already know that chemotherapy causes some side effects. The classic examples in movies and television are nausea and hair loss, but every regimen is different, and some regimens don't result in either of these side effects. Some side effects, such as nausea, can be controlled well with medication, while most—including hair loss—are temporary. Side effects such as nausea will change and improve in the days following an infusion, while other side effects may be cumulative over the course of a cycle of treatment.

The best way to prepare is to ask your oncologist what kinds of side effects are common for your regimen. Rather than asking for the entire list of possible side effects, ask for a list of the top three. Ask whether these side effects happen almost always, usually, or only sometimes. Ask how long these side effects are likely to last. You will also want to know whether any of the side effects can be cumulative. Will they likely be worst during the first infusions, or are they likely to be worst during the final infusions of a cycle? Whom do I call when something seems amiss or when I have a question? That last question is extremely important. Some oncologists will have you call an answering service, while others will give you an office number or their direct e-mail address or cell phone.

Knowing the answers to these questions will help you plan the other activities in your life, so that you are doing the things that are important to you when your energy is highest and when you feel most like yourself. Although side effects such as fatigue and nausea or rashes or mouth sores are disruptive and frustrating, there will likely be days during treatment when you feel pretty good. We talk a lot in treatment about planning to cope during those days when you feel crummy, but you also want to plan for those days when you feel strong and able to get out and live your life.

The most common side effects include fatigue, rash, diarrhea, hair loss, and mouth sores.

Fatigue. Most people experience fatigue in two ways. There is the immediate fatigue that a person feels after the infusion of chemotherapy. Some people fall asleep during the infusion. Most patients just hunker down those first couple days until they begin to feel better. The other kind of fatigue is more cumulative. If you are getting chemotherapy for several cycles, you may be more tired at the end of a cycle or at the end of several cycles.

Plan to get out and move around when you feel more energetic. Even going for a short walk will help you stay energized and keep you from becoming deconditioned, which can make you even more tired. We discuss fatigue more in chapter 16.

Rash. This is a common side effect of newer, targeted therapies. It looks sort of like an acne rash. One patient of mine was taking an oral regimen for chemotherapy, and she felt fine after each dose. The problem was that she had a rash on her face and that made her feel as though she didn't want anyone to see her. She told me that she felt like a fourteen-year-old kid and didn't want anyone taking pictures of her. We put her on an antibiotic for the rash, which cleared it up enough that she could go out without feeling that she had to explain why she looked so different.

Diarrhea. Certain therapies, including irinotecan, have this unfortunate side effect. The newer, targeted therapies can also cause bowel irritation. We discuss bowel-related side effects more in chapter 10, but the important thing to remember is to watch your diet. Some patients find that diarrhea is more stable when they take Imodium every day. One of my patients loved to eat salad, but it made her diarrhea worse. She found that she could eat salad once a week, and just plan to take more Imodium on that day. But you may find that there are certain foods that you can't eat while in treatment.

Hair loss. Remember that not all chemotherapy causes hair loss, and you'll have to ask your doctor whether you can expect this side effect. Thinning hair typically starts to be noticeable about three weeks after the beginning of a regimen. You may notice clumps of hair in the shower or on your pillow in the morning. Some regimens cause significant (short-term) hair loss, and you may want to keep a close-cropped haircut or even be fitted for a wig near the start of your treatment. Remember that it's temporary. Your hair will grow back, but this can feel like the first of many ways in which the cancer and its treatment change your body and your sense of self. You can read more about this aspect of living with cancer in chapter 8.

Mouth sores. One common side effect of chemotherapy is the tendency to get small mouth sores for a few days after infusion. This is often called mucositis (inflammation of the mucus membrane). Some chemotherapy regimens cause irritation in the mucus membranes inside the mouth, or sometimes they activate a previous herpes infection. These are a nuisance, although they typically heal quickly, but if they cause enough pain that you have trouble swallowing or opening your mouth or eating, you should contact your doctor.

Other Side Effects

Part II of this book details the most common ongoing side effects of treatment and how to manage them more effectively.

Some side effects can be permanent, and you will want to be informed about these as well. I recently had a patient who was an orthopedic surgeon. Cyndi loved operating, but her chemotherapy regimen came with a 20 percent chance of developing a permanent neuropathy (tingling or numbness in the hands and feet), which could affect her ability to operate. We could have chosen a less effective regimen that didn't have neuropathy as a side effect. In the end Cyndi decided to take her chances with the more effective regimen, and she thanked me for bringing it up as she started to mentally prepare for a life that might not include performing operations.

Planning Your Life after Infusions

Side effects tend to have a common rhythm. Many of my patients will say that they feel pretty crummy for the first two to three days immediately after the infusion. Many of them feel tired and sleep most of the first day after infusion. If the nausea is well controlled, they won't feel sick, but they won't feel like eating, either. Patients tend to feel better with each subsequent day after that until they are feeling much more like themselves. Depending on the structure of your cycle of chemotherapy, you may feel great for two weeks between infusions, or if you are on a weekly regimen, you might have only a few days that you feel like yourself.

Once you get a sense of how you are going to respond to a specific chemotherapy, you may decide a certain day is better for the infusion. Some people like infusions early in the week so they are feeling better by the weekend, while others like the infusions later in the week so they can hunker down over the weekend and then feel better during the week. One of my patients was a nurse who loved her job so much that she didn't want to stop working while being treated for stage 4 ovarian cancer. She didn't want to stay home the week after her infusions. She found that she preferred to get each infusion on a Friday, so that she could deal with fatigue over the weekend. By Tuesday, she would feel good enough to return to work, although she still needed rest times during the day. She was able to schedule her shifts so that she had a longer break at lunch and could rest for a couple of hours in the middle of the day that first week. By the second week after each infusion, she felt good enough to resume her usual work schedule.

There are no right or wrong answers. Just think about what might work best for you, and know that the clinic should be able to adapt to the schedule you prefer.

Additional Support

Starting treatment is always challenging, and more often cancer centers are including supportive services to help you relieve stress and ease into the cadence of chemotherapy. These might include massage, acupuncture, music or art therapy, or time with a social worker or religious counselor. Your palliative care team and your infusion nurses will be a great source for additional therapies available both inside the cancer clinic and within the community.

Chemo Holidays

Everybody needs a break sometimes, even in the middle of a chemotherapy regimen. You may have an important trip planned or a family gathering for which you want to feel as much like yourself as possible. Many people benefit from having a little time away from chemotherapy. You can always discuss the option of delaying a treatment to accommodate a life event or special trip. These delays are often called chemo holidays, and oncologists understand that cancer treatment is one part of your life, but not your whole life. You should be able to take a break if you need one.

For those patients on lifelong chemotherapy, these breaks in treatment can be wonderful, even if not tied to a specific event. Some are extended breaks from treatment that last for several months. This will give you some time to feel normal again without having to spend time in the infusion unit. If you are receiving lifelong chemotherapy, you should definitely ask about the possibility of a chemo holiday. If you have a curable cancer, there may be excellent reasons why your doctor will not want you to take a break from chemo.

Fertility and Chemotherapy

Going through chemotherapy can affect your fertility, and if you are concerned about remaining fertile after treatment, you will want to talk to your doctor about how your body may be affected by treatment. Some women harvest eggs and some men bank sperm before starting chemotherapy. You want to think about the future if having children is a priority for you.

How Chemotherapy Affects the Family

One of the unpredictable side effects of chemotherapy is how it affects the whole family. Whether it's your spouse, children, parents, or siblings, people will react differently to your chemotherapy because they want to help but don't know how. These are incredibly stressful times for families. Everyone wants to do the right thing, but some things are more helpful than others. I am going to list some of the tricky issues that come up for patients and families. They may or may not apply to you.

- Your family is pushing you, thinking there is something wrong with you because you feel really tired the week you get chemotherapy. They are forever pushing you to do more than you feel you can.
- You have a mile-long list of phone calls from people who want to visit to "keep your spirits up" during treatment. You are not sure you want to see all these people when you are feeling sick.
- Your loved ones push you to eat when you are not hungry after chemotherapy and worry that you are "giving up."
- After a visit with the oncology team, everyone in your family wants an update. It is exhausting.
- Your loved ones are able to come only intermittently. When they do, they ask all kinds of questions about matters you have already discussed with them. It feels like they don't believe that you are telling the truth about what the doctors have said.

Over the years, I have found some things help treatment go more smoothly. First, have one or two people who come to all of your appointments (or as many appointments as possible). One of them should be the agent of your health care proxy. This is crucial. You need to designate a person to make medical decisions for you if you are too sick to make them yourself. This person should be present for nearly every appointment so that he or she hears the same information that you are hearing. It is also important to talk about your wishes for treatments with this person.

During these appointments your loved ones have the opportunity to ask as many questions as they like. You can encourage a discussion about any of the issues they have been bugging you about. Sometimes it is helpful for them to hear the same message from your team that you are telling them. Sometimes they will want more or less information than you want to hear. This is normal. Your spouse or your sister might want to know everything about what might happen if treatment doesn't go as well as we hope, and you may not. Or you might want to know about what might happen if the cancer progresses, while they want to hear nothing about it. Your medical team knows that you get to decide how much information you want to have about the future. And you can work with your team to get everyone's needs met.

I had a patient, Rick, who wanted to know as much information about the future as possible while his wife was feeling particularly overwhelmed and didn't want to think about anything but the current treatments. I would meet with the family at first, and then when Rick had additional questions, he and his daughter would stay to talk with Dave and me while his wife went for coffee.

You may have a larger group of people you want to meet the oncology team as well. It is fine to talk to your oncologist about having periodic family meetings so everyone can ask their questions. These often make sense when it is time to change to a new chemotherapy.

These family meetings are different from the clinic appointments that take place on the day of each infusion. Your infusion-day appointments become fairly routine after a while. It might be nice to have someone with you to pass the time, or it may be necessary to have someone drive you home if you are feeling crummy, but in the appointments before each infusion, your doctor will not usually be providing new information about how the treatments are working. For those appointments when your doctor will be reviewing scans or talking about treatment options, you may want to invite different people to join you, so that everyone hears the same information at the same time.

6

Tests and Scans in Treatment

ONE OF THE FIRST THINGS you learn in treatment is that you're going to be subjected to a lot of tests. That's one of the reasons your appointments with your oncologist are going to be rushed. It's not just the oncologist who has a tight schedule. You will have one, too. You have to get blood work done every time, and you have to get to the pharmacy to get the chemo drugs, and you have to get to the infusion unit where you will spend between two and eight hours. On some days you'll also have scans. The results of these tests may cause significant changes in your treatment regimen, and if you know why these tests are done and what the results mean, you can better understand what's happening in your body and what your medical team is telling you.

For example, the other day I was paged to the infusion unit where a patient was waiting to get chemo. Libby is in her midsixties and she is at the end of her first cycle of chemo for esophageal cancer. She's on the board of several museums and arts organizations, and she's always impeccably dressed. She sometimes talks to me less like a doctor and more like a favorite nephew who could use a little advice. She's forever handing me Xeroxes of news stories I ought to have read about health care reform and if there is a smudge on my tie, she will find it. In other words, we get along great.

But that day I had to deliver some unsettling news. She wasn't going to be able to get chemotherapy until the following week because her blood counts were too low. I told her that I hoped her blood counts would rise by the following week, and if so, she could take chemo again. This is not an uncommon occurrence in cancer treatment. Sometimes a symptom that is a side effect of the chemotherapy will cause us to alter the treatment regimen. As Vicki mentioned in the previous chapter, we want to provide cancer treatment to patients in a manner that is safe, effective, and allows for the best quality of life that is possible. I think all oncologists strive for this.

She was disappointed, of course. When you've mentally prepared for an infusion and set aside your whole day for it, you are going to be disappointed if it doesn't happen. Libby also worried aloud that this delay would derail her progress. I explained that this isn't the case. One week off isn't likely to change her prognosis, but giving chemo when blood counts are low is dangerous. In fact, one reason I was visiting Libby was to ask a lot of follow-up questions about how she was feeling. Did she have a fever or chills? Was she fatigued? How was her appetite? What we don't want to happen is for the low blood counts to mask an infection that your body can't adequately fight. This is why blood tests are so crucial.

Blood Tests

Blood tests are going to be a big part of your life as a cancer patient. You will likely have blood drawn every time you come to the clinic. You might hate the idea of having blood taken, and I don't blame you. While many nurses and technicians are experts at finding a vein and slipping the needle in painlessly, not everyone can do this every time. If you've had a portacath placed under your skin for infusions, ask the nurse to draw the blood through that instead of your skin. Sure, it takes a few minutes, but for most people it's painless every time and will keep you from feeling like a pin cushion.

There are three main categories of blood tests that your oncologist will order: counts, chemistries, and tumor markers.

Blood Counts

Every time you have your blood drawn, the lab will do a complete blood count (CBC). This measures the three main types of blood cells that your bone marrow makes:

- *White blood cells.* This is the army of immune soldiers that fight infection in your system. When your white blood count is low, you are prone to serious infection and can rapidly get very sick without knowing it.
- *Red blood cells.* These carry oxygen around your body. When the red blood count is low, you have anemia and are more prone to fatigue and breathlessness.
- *Platelets.* These help the blood to clot, and if you have a low platelet count, you are more prone to bleeding, including internal bleeding.

White Blood Cells

There are two broad categories of white blood cells: myeloid cells and lymphocytes. Counting the myeloid cells is crucial because these are the ones that fight off bacteria, something your body is doing all day, every day. I hate to be the first one to tell you this, but you have bacteria all over your body. Your skin, respiratory tract, and your gastrointestinal (GI) tract all have bacteria living in and on them as part of their natural function. Your blood cells know how to keep bacteria in check. There is a specific subcategory of myeloid cell—called a neutrophil—that is the first line of defense against bacterial invaders in the body. Neutrophils keep bacteria at the proper level and keep them from entering the bloodstream. In fact, neutrophils actually look like strange little Pac-Men under the microscope. (And if you want to sound nerdy to your oncologist, you can refer to these cells as "polys," which is short for polymorphonuclear.)

You need a lot of neutrophils to stay healthy and alive, because if bacteria get into the bloodstream, you can get very sick, often over a matter of hours. This used to be called blood poisoning, but now doctors use terms such as sepsis or bacteremia, and it is a medical emergency. If your absolute neutrophil count goes below 1,000, then you are at risk for developing bacteria in the bloodstream (more about infection in chapter 14).

Your CBC will report the number of neutrophils first as a percentage of your total white blood cells (for example, 25 percent of 2,000 WBCs). Most lab slips will do the work for you and multiply the percentage by the total white blood cells and give you the absolute neutrophil count, or ANC (ANC 500 in the example above). Oncologists are obsessed with ANCs, and sadly you will probably come to share this obsession. We usually don't offer chemotherapy unless the ANC is at a certain level—usually above 1,000. If your doctor is concerned about your dropping ANC, he or she may suggest something called growth factor support. Growth factors are naturally occurring proteins that your body uses to boost the cell count. Drug companies have figured out how to make them (Neupogen and Neulasta are two common ones), and your doctor can administer them to you after you get chemotherapy.

Your CBC will also contain a count for the second type of white blood cell, a lymphocyte. These are the generals of the immune system because they direct all the other white blood cells in attacking an infection. While they are less important than neutrophils on a day-to-day basis, they are the core of your immune system. For example, a T-cell, which is attacked in HIV infections, is a type of lymphocyte. The good news is that most chemotherapy drugs don't affect the lymphocytes to a significant degree. Some people, particularly those with liquid tumors such as leukemia or lymphoma, can have significant problems because their lymphocytes get too low or don't function effectively because of the presence of the lymphoma or leukemia. People with low- or poor-functioning lymphocytes can get multiple infections, often with uncommon bacteria or viruses, so-called opportunistic infections. Sometimes patients with solid tumors can get opportunistic infections because they have had high doses of steroids (such as prednisone and dexamethasone) with their chemotherapy. One of the many side effects of steroids is that it decreases the effectiveness of lymphocytes and puts people at risk for opportunistic infections.

If your lymphocyte count gets too low, below 200 for example, your oncologist will give you strategies to help protect you against infections. Often patients with low lymphocyte counts have to be on prophylactic antibiotics. Your doctors may also have to change the way that they use steroids with your chemotherapy.

Red Blood Cells

Your oncologist is going to be watching your red blood cell count (RBC) to see whether you have anemia. Both the cancer and the chemotherapy will inhibit your bone marrow's ability to make red blood cells. If cancer is the cause, we call it anemia of chronic disease, and if chemotherapy is the cause, we call it chemotherapy-induced anemia. Radiation can also cause anemia by damaging your bone marrow where the red blood cells are made. Surgery can cause anemia too, either through direct blood loss at the time of surgery or if your surgery has removed portions of your bowel that aid in absorbing iron or vitamin B12, two essential nutrients in red blood cell development. These causes don't have to be a big concern. Your oncologist will have seen low RBC numbers many times before. In fact, you probably won't have any symptoms from anemia unless your RBC, or hematocrit, falls below 30. If it does, your doctor may recommend either blood transfusions or an injectable medication designed to boost your bone marrow production of RBC. Each approach has its advantages and disadvantages, which you can discuss with your doctor.

If you do have low RBC, or develop it quickly, your doctor may ask questions or do some tests to see whether the anemia might be caused by internal bleeding, rather than the cancer or the chemotherapy. For example, my patients with stomach cancer or colon cancer sometimes have tumors that bleed into the GI tract. You can easily tell if you have been passing blood from the colon because you will see bright red blood mixed with your stool. If the bleeding occurs higher in the GI tract—in the stomach or esophagus—the blood will turn a dark black color and you'll see what looks like tar mixed with your stool. That's why your doctor will ask you if your stool looks dark and tarry. If you notice this at home, or if you notice bright red blood in your stool, you should contact your doctor right away. Internal bleeding sounds scary, but there's usually a solution. You might be admitted to the hospital to undergo a lower or upper endoscopy to figure out where the blood is coming from. Once the source has been found, your doctor may recommend surgery, radiation, chemotherapy, or embolization, which is a procedure that blocks the source of the bleeding (more about bleeding in chapter 15).

If you have hematologic malignancies such as lymphoma or leukemia, you may be anemic because something is destroying your red blood cells. Oncologists call this a consumptive or hemolytic process. Cancer sometimes makes an antibody against the red blood cells, which destroys them. It's rare in solid tumors, but possible. Your doctor may suggest steroids in addition to the anticancer drugs to calm down the immune system that is attacking your red blood cells.

Blood Chemistries

After counting the number and type of cells in your blood sample, the lab will test for chemical compounds found in your blood. We call these results the blood chemistries, and there are three results your doctor will be looking at: electrolytes, kidney function, and liver function. These tests should be ordered for you at every visit to the clinic in which you get an infusion, and the lab will need about forty-five minutes to return the results. You usually won't be allowed to get chemotherapy if the numbers don't look good, so you should expect to arrive at the clinic at least forty-five minutes before your scheduled infusion to get your blood drawn and your labs started.

Electrolytes are minerals in your system, and they are often part of a blood screening because they are markers of health, such as the proper balance of hydration, and an electrolyte imbalance can be an early sign of a developing problem. Your oncologist will be looking at your levels of sodium (NA), potassium (K), magnesium (MG), and calcium (CA). When these are too high or too low, doctors know to look further, because you might be sick without realizing it. The good news is that it's often an easy fix.

For example, Margot was a patient of mine with bile duct cancer. She saw an oncologist in her community two hours outside of Boston but would come see me every other month for additional consultations. At one appointment she told me she was feeling run down and tired and that this was a different kind of tired than she'd ever felt from chemotherapy. She was worried that the cancer was getting worse. Even her oncologist called me and told me that he thought the cancer was getting worse, although the scans didn't show it. I asked Margot to get some CT scans, and they showed that the cancer looked stable. But when I saw her I could tell that she wasn't the same person. She had no energy and looked defeated. When her labs came back, I saw that her calcium level was very elevated, over 11. We figured out that her tumor was now making a protein that mimicked parathyroid hormone, which is a hormone that regulates calcium homeostasis. When you have too much parathyroid hormone, your calcium can get too high and you get extremely tired. When I first started practicing in the early 1990s, this was a huge problem in cancer clinics. At the time, the only treatment we had was giving the patient fluids. Now, there is a class of drugs called bisphosphonates that can bring the calcium into the normal range within hours and keep it there. We gave it to Margot, and she felt better that same day.

Kidney function is a critical marker for your doctor to monitor during treatment. Many of the drugs that you take are filtered out over time and eliminated by the kidneys. If your kidneys aren't functioning well to filter your blood, certain medications can accumulate in the bloodstream and become toxic. This is particularly true of chemotherapy drugs. Kidney (renal) function tests include the blood urea nitrogen and the creatinine. Usually your blood urea nitrogen is less than 20 and your creatinine is less than 1.0. If these are abnormal, your doctor will look into it right away and may even delay your next infusion. Many times, there is an easy explanation for an abnormal kidney function. It could be something as simple as dehydration caused by one of the chemotherapy drugs, and we can eliminate the problem by eliminating that one drug. Sometimes cancers block the ureters, the tubes that carry urine from the kidneys, and cause kidney dysfunction. Whatever the reason, your oncologist will be paying close attention to these numbers.

In addition to electrolytes and kidney function, your doctor will be looking at your liver function tests (LFTs). You may already know that the liver carries out the vital function of clearing the blood of toxins, but it also makes many of the necessary proteins for the body.

These proteins are created in the hepatocytes, the main cells of the liver. If those cells are damaged, they will release enzymes into the blood that can be measured in the lab. So your doctor is going to be looking at something called aspartate aminotransferase (AST, once known as SGOT) and alanine aminotransferase (ALT, sometimes called SGPT). When these numbers go up, doctors usually suspect inflammation of the liver caused by chemotherapy drugs. An elevated level can also mean that there are cancer cells active in the liver. What you need to know is that your doctor may be reluctant to give more chemotherapy in the short term when those levels go up. He or she may be concerned that your liver cells won't be able to effectively filter the drug out of your system, which means you would be at risk for developing toxic levels of the drug in your blood.

Your liver also makes bile that gets secreted through the biliary tree down into the small intestine. And, yes, the lab will be conducting special screenings for this function as well. An elevated alkaline phosphatase (ALP, or alk phos) level reveals damage to cells near the bile ducts. Bilirubin is actually a yellowish substance in the bile, and if the duct is blocked, that substance will build up in your bloodstream. When you have way too much of it in your system, your skin and the whites of your eyes will actually turn yellow.

Chemotherapy drugs are also eliminated through the biliary system, and so your doctor will want to investigate any elevated levels of ALP and bilirubin. You may be asked to get a CT scan looking for dilated bile ducts, which would indicate that something is blocking the ducts. In that case, you will probably have to have what we call an endoscopic retrograde cholangiopancreatography (ERCP). This is a procedure that would require sedation while the gastroenterologist threads a thin tube down through the esophagus, the stomach, and into the first part of the small intestine, looking for that blockage. If the blocked duct is visible, the doctor will insert a metal or plastic tube (stent), which is a lot like the coronary stents used to prop open arteries, across the obstruction to keep the duct open. That may sound intimidating, but it's more common than you think. Many patients with cancers of the GI tract have had more than one ERCP to implant stents to keep bile ducts open and functioning.

Tumor Markers

Cancer cells are constantly producing proteins that get secreted into the bloodstream. Lab technicians can measure the levels of those proteins, and the result is what we call tumor markers. In general, the more cancer cells you have, the higher the tumor markers in your blood. As the number of cancer cells decreases, the marker numbers go down.

The whole subject of tumor markers can be confusing. First, scientists are all the time discovering new ones and figuring out what the measurements might mean. Second, not all cancers with the same markers produce the same level of that marker. So, you can't compare your tumor marker to your neighbor's. Your tumor markers are specific to your cancer alone. Third, even normal tissues can produce these markers. At this point, you may be wondering why doctors bother to follow these numbers.

On the one hand, if you've had a tumor removed by a surgeon, your specific tumor markers should return to normal. Your doctor is going to follow markers in your blood tests to see if they go up again, which might mean that the cancer has returned. If they go up, you will probably want to get some scans, either CT, PET, or MRI (discussed below), to see whether there are visible tumors.

On the other hand, if you have metastatic cancer, meaning that you have tumors in multiple sites in your body, your doctor will monitor the tumor markers to see how the treatment is working. When those levels go down over time, we suspect that the tumors are getting smaller or that there are fewer cancerous cells circulating in your body. While the reduction of tumor markers is a great sign, your doctor will always order scans to confirm the result.

I have a lot of patients who are engineers and they sometimes like to make charts and even statistical analyses for aspects of their blood work. These charts look really cool and interesting, and they often show weekly fluctuations in tumor markers, which the patient then wants me to explain. Unfortunately, tumor markers do change week to week—even day to day—but those small changes don't actually signal anything. Cells generate more or less of these proteins based on many factors. Tumor markers correlate only generally to the tumor burden in your body and aren't a specific measurement of the tumors themselves.

Scans

Ask anyone about life with cancer and inevitably the conversation will come around to scans. This is the primary way you and your doctor will follow your progress and see how your treatment is working.

Scans are radiology studies that image your body. They include computed tomography (CT), positron emission tomography (PET), and magnetic resonance imaging (MRI). These are the same scans doctors used to diagnose your cancer.

Now that you are in treatment, you'll be having scans about every two to three months, and you will need to review those scans with your doctor a day or two after they have been taken. Waiting for scan results can be distressing, and you want to shorten your wait as much as possible. Some patients tell me waiting for scan results is a kind of torture. Don't accept torture. Make sure you schedule an appointment with your oncologist first, and then schedule the scan for the day before. That way you have just one day to wait, and you know that when you see your oncologist the scans will be ready and you can look at them and talk about them together.

Many patients beg me to call them and go over the scans by phone. I almost always insist that they come into the clinic. The biggest mistakes of my career have happened when I violated this rule. In these cases, I failed to communicate the findings effectively, the patient failed to understand what I was saying, or I failed to understand the questions the patient was asking. I've learned the hard way that telephone calls leave too much to abstract description. You and your doctor want to be able to point to spots on the scans while you are discussing them. These can be some of the most meaningful and important conversations you have with your oncologist because they will lead to detailed discussions about prognosis and treatment. Don't do it by phone.

It may be tempting to think that your oncologist will call you or schedule an appointment with you to go over the scans you've just had taken. But that probably won't happen. Remember that your on-cologist may be treating several hundred active patients. Most clinics don't circulate printed reports between departments. Everything is stored in a database. When you get a scan, the radiologist will study it and generate a report, and, unless that report shows a potential emergency, it will sit there until the oncologist reviews it. That's why having a scheduled appointment at the clinic is the best way to get immediate news about your scans.

Also, make sure your oncologist has reviewed your scans with the radiologist. Scans are tricky to interpret, and if your oncologist is just reading the radiologist's report, he or she may have missed some of the subtleties. Your doctor knows everything about how you are feeling, and the radiologist knows everything about what the scans say, so make sure they have talked to each other about the scans. This conversation is the chance for your doctor to ask important follow-up questions about what the radiologist has seen.

For example, I had a patient with colon cancer that was starting to metastasize. His wife had called me the morning of our scheduled appointment to say that the patient had developed terrible pain in his neck. This was new. I grabbed his scans, and, sure enough, there was what looked like a lesion on his spine at the base of his neck. Was this an instance of bone metastasis? I couldn't tell. So I asked a radiologist to call up the scans taken the day before. She scrolled over the pictures of his spine and within a few seconds said, "No. It's a slipped disc." I was so relieved but had to ask, "Are you sure?" She gave me such a look of disdain. Radiologists are absolute experts at reading scans. Although they aren't always this sure about what a scan shows or whether a scan shows progress, they know more about scans than anyone in the hospital. She scrolled over it again, slowly for my benefit, and then said she was sure.

Computerized Tomography (CT) Scans

These are the most common scans ordered by doctors. The scans take thousands of pictures of your body in slices, and then sophisticated software reconstructs those slices into a three-dimensional whole. You may have had one of these scans during the process of diagnosing your cancer, and the subsequent scans will be similar.

A CT scan is most helpful in tracking cancer when there is some kind of contrast in the body, a substance that highlights blood vessels and makes more tumors visible, which are often more vascular than the surrounding tissue. With intravenous contrast, doctors can more easily see tumors in your body because they will help outline the areas of cancer on the scan. There are two types of contrasts, oral and IV.

Patients getting a scan of the abdomen may be asked to take an oral contrast, something you drink before the scan, which outlines the GI tract and makes it easier to distinguish these organs from other tissues. The oral contrast may cause some cramping and diarrhea, and if it does, you should stop taking it. The truth is that oral contrast isn't critical to reading most scans. IV contrast, however, is extremely important, and it should be given in most instances.

The problem with IV contrast is that some people begin to develop allergies to it, and if that happens, doctors worry that it can lead to anaphylactic shock. You'll know you are developing an allergy if you get an itchy feeling after the IV starts or develop hives on your skin. In that case, we may have to administer steroids before the IV contrast. Sometimes the steroids are effective in controlling the allergy, but sometimes people can't tolerate the IV contrast, and it needs to be omitted. The IV contrast may also not be appropriate for people with poor kidney function, because it can lead to kidney failure. These are some reasons your doctor may omit the IV contrast before your scan.

Reading CT Scans

When you look at a CT scan, the different images may not look like much of anything to you, but your doctor can point out the bones and different organs and can scroll through each slice to show you the outlines of visible tumors. A tumor needs to be about five millimeters in size to be visible. If it is any smaller, it will blend into the surrounding tissue. Yet that tiny five-millimeter tumor will still contain about one billion cancer cells. People are astounded to learn that they can have a collection of one hundred million cancer cells in a tumor that is still too small to detect on a scan. That's why doctors order scans throughout treatment. This is the only way we can see whether something is growing or shrinking.

Doctors use all kinds of terms to describe cancer: nodule, mass, tumor, lesion. It's easy to get hung up on these words, but they all mean cancer. Sometimes it's easy to follow the progress of cancer with CT scans. A lemon-sized lesion can become orange sized, or it can shrink down to the size of a walnut. If progress is slower, we can still put calipers around lesions and measure them accurately. But it's not always so straightforward. Some cancer spreads less like a discrete mass and more like a moss that grows along the planes of a tissue, making it difficult to tell the normal tissue from the cancer. Peritoneal carcinomatosis, which grows in the abdomen, spreads more like grains of sand, and this can be hard to track even though it wreaks havoc with the GI system (see chapter 10).

Positron Emission Tomography (PET) Scans

PET scans are nuclear medicine scans. A radiologist injects a radioactive isotope into the veins and then can detect where that substance accumulates. For a PET scan, radiologists usually use something called fluorodeoxyglucose, which is a glucose-based dye that is taken up readily by metabolically active tissues such as cancer.

Patients will often insist that they get PET scans because they think that PET scans are better than CT scans. But that's not always the case. PET scans are well suited for following some cancers like lymphomas. They can also be very useful for the initial workup of certain cancers such as lung cancer. However, they don't give good spatial resolution so they are often combined with a CT scan, and these scans are called PET-CTs. The CT portion of a PET-CT is often a noncontrast CT with nondiagnostic quality. The CT is just good enough for us to be able to note where the fluorodeoxyglucose is being accumulated.

Except for lymphomas, if I had to pick one test to follow a cancer, I would always choose a contrast-enhanced CT scan over a PET scan.

Magnetic Resonance Imaging (MRI)

An MRI uses magnetic fields and radio waves to form images of the body. The radiologist may also use a contrast agent called gadolinium, which is generally safe unless you have poor kidney function. These tests are much better than CT scans at imaging a particular organ but worse when you need to scan a whole section of the body such as the chest or abdomen. The most common reason for getting an MRI is to get an image of the brain, spinal cord, and liver because the MRI does a better job of finding metastases in these areas.

As a patient, you may prefer a CT scan, because the MRI requires you to go into the tube and hold still for up to an hour. This can be distressing if you suffer from claustrophobia or have trouble holding one position because of pain. You can take antianxiety medications such as lorazepam or pain medications such as morphine before getting an MRI.

MRIs are read in a fashion similar to CTs. Compared with CTs, MRIs have slightly better resolution of a particular organ. For instance, MRIs of the brain and the liver can show metastases when CTs completely miss them. Patrick was a sixty-two-year-old man with metastatic lung cancer, who was admitted to the hospital with balance difficulties. The emergency room had done a CT scan that didn't show anything. The doctors in the emergency room had decided to admit him anyway because they were concerned about him. After a few hours of hydration, Patrick was feeling better and wanted to go home, but we convinced him to stay and get an MRI. The MRI showed a two-centimeter brain metastasis in his cerebellum, the part of the brain that controls balance. We had the neurosurgeon see him right away, and later that afternoon the surgeon removed the brain metastasis. The next morning Patrick was feeling great and walking the halls without any difficulty.

Scan Results

In general, there are only three results that a scan will show while you are in treatment. First, it could show that the cancer is responding to treatment and the tumors are getting smaller. Second, the scan could show that things are basically the same, which means that the cancer is still responding to treatment. The third possibility is that the scan shows that the cancer is advancing.

If you are in a phase of treatment that doctors call surveillance or follow-up, then the doctor will generally be concerned only about the third possibility, that the cancer is active again. If there is no change during follow-up, the doctor will say, "Your scans look fine," which essentially means that everything is the same.

Unfortunately, sometimes doctors aren't sure whether things are better, worse, or the same, which can be extremely unnerving. We all want definitive news. Doctors want to be able to tell patients exactly what's going on and how well the treatment is working, and it's so easy for doctors and patients alike to feel frustrated by all the uncertainty. Remember that a scan can read a tumor only if it is at least a half centimeter wide, so it's possible that your body contains tumors the scan can't yet read. A scan can also show something that looks like a tumor but isn't.

One of the most common causes of uncertainty are little spots on the lung called pulmonary nodules. They are too small to biopsy and too small to really identify. Doctors often refer to them as "ditzels." About half of all adults have them, and they are perfectly normal. But in cancer patients, we worry that one or more of them might be a metastasis of the primary cancer. We can follow these ditzels on scan after scan, and they usually don't grow or change, but sometimes they do. In fact, there are many findings on scans that are most likely benign but that we are obligated to follow once we find them.

Sometimes, patients and doctors worry that the radiation exposure from all the scans will put them at risk to develop more cancer. Each CT scan of the chest or abdomen gives you the same amount of radiation that you receive from general background radiation over the course of two to three years. Over many years, too much exposure to radiation can raise your risk of developing certain kinds of cancers, particularly cancers of the bone marrow like leukemia and myelodysplastic syndrome. Usually the risk of not following one of these small, indeterminate nodules is greater than the theoretically minute risk of getting a radiation-induced cancer.

Other Tests Your Doctor May Ask For

Your oncologist may want you to undergo tests on your DNA, or your genetics, in part to see whether your cancer has a genetic basis and therefore the risk of developing cancer could be shared by other members of your family. These tests are optional, but doctors tend to suggest them when a cancer patient is under the age of fifty or if there are multiple first-degree relatives (mother, father, siblings, children) with cancer in the family.

Cancer is disease of genes, or DNA, and it develops because of an accumulation of mutations in the DNA. I like to use the illustration that a cancer cell is like a runaway train. It may run rampant because the accelerator stays on until it overcomes the braking mechanism of the train. Or the braking mechanism is faulty, so the train can't slow down or stop when it needs to. Perhaps the mechanic is incompetent and eventually the accelerating mechanism and braking mechanisms come into disrepair during normal cell division. Most cancers are due to accumulated mutations in the accelerator, braking, or mechanical parts of the genome.

The genes that you are born with are called your germ-line genes. Mutations occur in your germ-line genes that you inherited from your mom (egg) or dad (sperm). Mutations also occur in your germ-line genes de novo, meaning that your mom or dad didn't have them, but they occurred in the formation of the egg or sperm. Either way, some of these mutations can put you at risk for developing cancer at a young age.

Inherited forms of cancer are due to inherited mutations in the germ-line DNA that are in accelerator genes, the braking genes, or the genes responsible for repairing mistakes during cell division. One of the most common inherited germ-line mutations are the BRCA (pronounced "bracka") mutations that put women at risk for breast and ovarian cancer and men at risk for prostate and pancreatic cancer (among others). There are two main types of mutations, called BRCA1 and BRCA2, that carry different risks for different cancers. The BRCA genes are called tumor-suppressor genes and are part of that braking mechanism that the cell uses. Women who have BRCA mutations are at risk for cancers in both breasts and their ovaries.

So if we diagnose a young woman with a BRCA gene mutation, this will not only affect the risk of cancer potentially in her sisters, brothers, and children; it may also affect how we approach her cancer. Rather than undergoing a lumpectomy to remove her breast cancer, she may want to consider bilateral mastectomy and reconstruction so that she doesn't have to worry about developing a cancer in her other breast.

There are a number of inherited predispositions to cancer for which we may ask you to undergo testing. These tests are different from the molecular pathology tests (described in chapter 2) where we look at the mutations that are specific to your cancer and driving the cancer through the malignant process, which we call somatic mutations to distinguish them from germ-line mutations.

7

How Am I Supposed to Cope with This?

A DIAGNOSIS OF SERIOUS CANCER can affect every area of your life, and the busier and more active you were before your diagnosis, the more you can feel that your life has been derailed, and the more coping strategies you are going to need to get yourself back on track. Jane was in her late forties when she was diagnosed with metastatic colon cancer. Before her diagnosis, she was in the middle of an MBA program that she started after her two kids went off to college, and she was an avid skier and hiker who spent most weekends hiking the woods of western Massachusetts with her dog. She had been hoping to earn her graduate degree and go back to work full time.

One day, I asked her how she was doing with her daily life, and she said, "I can't believe how much has changed in three months. Everything has been taken over by treatments. I can't do any of the things I love to do. I don't know how to make any plans for the future."

This feeling is completely normal. What Jane needed and what all newly diagnosed patients need is a plan B, along with some strategies for coping with these overwhelming feelings. This starts with figuring out what's important to you and what you can do given your health status and energy level.

Jane thought about what was important to her. She knew that her energy was lower than normal and that she wanted to use the energy she did have for her boys, who frequently came home from college to see her. She decided to quit her MBA program, but she also wanted to do something that brought meaning to her life. She started volunteering in the office of the local animal shelter. She had to figure out how to be out in the woods even if she didn't feel up to doing her usual five-mile hike. She had to find foods to eat other than the salads she loved because they made her diarrhea worse.

Many people feel powerless in the first months after diagnosis. It's tempting to feel that your life has ended, but it hasn't. Your life isn't what you had envisioned, but you can adapt. You can learn how to live with the cancer. You have the power to be engaged with what's happening and make your life the best it can be.

Learning to cope effectively while living with a new cancer diagnosis means having a safe place to talk about the ways in which the cancer has changed your life while finding ways to stay engaged in the world. Social workers can be very helpful with this. A palliative care clinician can help you strategize about how to set goals and manage energy and other symptoms so you can do more of what you want. In this chapter I'll describe coping strategies that will make it easier to get through each day.

Why Me?

It is normal to look for something or someone to blame. You may be feeling that your health choices or lifestyle choices may have led you to this point. Patients often ask their doctors whether they did something to cause the cancer. The short answer is no. Although, technically, individuals can put themselves at an increased risk of getting cancer through certain behaviors, there is no direct line between a particular behavior and definitely getting cancer. Not everyone who smokes gets lung cancer, and some people get lung cancer even though they never smoked. A big part of cancer is just dumb luck. Your cancer diagnosis is not a punishment for past behavior, nor is it a punishment for failing to get certain health screenings.

Ultimately, cancer is a biological process and mostly beyond your control. I stress this because I have had patients who insist that their impeccable health choices should have exempted them from cancer. People say to me, "I run five miles a day. I drink kale smoothies. I meditate. I'm kind to animals. How can this be happening?" And I get it. You want your terrific health choices to count for something. Secretly, you maybe want them to transform themselves into a "get out of jail free" card for cancer. This is a kind of wishful thinking, and while it's normal for these thoughts to cross your mind from time to time, you don't want to cling to them. Over time, this belief that you ought to have a special health status will drain your energy. It's similar to the belief that some people have that they will be cured as long as they only think positive thoughts. Oncologists sometimes call this "the tyranny of optimism," because this belief becomes so exhausting for patients and their families and yet is so pervasive in the larger culture.

You can waste a lot of energy telling yourself that you deserve a certain outcome in treatment because you never smoked or never ate meat or never missed a workout. But, in reality, the best course of action now is to engage with a good treatment team and make a good plan to treat the cancer.

Coping Doesn't Mean Fighting

In the larger culture people often refer to coping with cancer as a battle and the illness as something that must be fought if it is ever going to be defeated. In some ways this is a comforting metaphor for any serious illness, because you can cast the illness as the villain and yourself as the hero who will fight at all costs. If you are supporting someone who has cancer, you may use this metaphor because it means that all of your sacrifices and hard work are part of this critical battle. But this metaphor has limitations, specifically because it stresses that dealing with cancer ultimately divides patients into winners and losers. If the treatments work well and the tumors shrink, it's great to feel like a winner. But what if the biology of the cancer doesn't allow for this? You are not a loser if your cancer advances.

Having worked with thousands of patients, I can tell you that the patients who cope best in this new world of cancer treatment are the ones who give up on the notion that they can push the cancer away by fighting it, being tough enough, or by enduring treatments and side effects stoically.

The most successful patients come to feel that cancer is a kind of partner in their lives. That may sound strange, because of course you would never have chosen cancer as a partner or wished it on anyone else. But altering your metaphor from a battle to a partnership allows you to spend your energy working around the cancer and all of the changes it has brought to your life. You can try to enjoy what's going on in your life in spite of treatments. You may want to find ways to celebrate or treat yourself on the days when you feel most energetic. Later on, you may be surprised to find that cancer has altered your life in positive ways as well.

One of my patients with lung cancer, whom I had been seeing for about eighteen months, confessed to me that he had never felt closer to his adult children as he had during treatment. Both of his children lived busy lives on the other side of the country and had the habit of coming home only briefly on major holidays. Since his diagnosis, they used their vacations and family leave to come home and stay with him for weeks at a time. He did perfectly ordinary things with them, fixing dinner, watching baseball games on TV, gardening, but for him these were treasured times, a chance to reconnect with his kids as a dad and as a person. "This would never have happened if I didn't have cancer," he told me. That is not to say that he liked having cancer. He didn't. But he was able to appreciate that it had brought new focus and urgency to his family relationships.

Symptom Management

The first step in effective coping is to make sure you can talk to your doctor about your symptoms and any side effects of the cancer treatment itself. It's going to be harder to make plans for doing things you love and finding ways to cope emotionally if you are undertreating any pain that you have or if your doctor doesn't know that you have neuropathy (numbness or pain in your hands and feet) or nausea or bowel troubles. I urge patients to keep a daily diary of symptoms and reactions to medications. Your oncologist is undoubtedly busy and probably focused on tests and scans and trying to make sure your chemotherapy regimen is working the way it should. Plan to bring a list of your top three symptom concerns to each visit and ask how your medical team can help you with them.

Using Multiple Strategies

Like Jane, many people use physical activity as a way to stay fit and also as a way to discharge stress. You may have enjoyed running or swimming or lifting weights as a way to calm down and feel centered. You can certainly modify your workouts to do them for as long as possible. I've worked with patients who loved yoga, and together we modified poses for them to do on those days when they were dealing with fatigue or pain. There will likely be times during your treatment when your favorite fitness activities are difficult or no longer possible. Exceptionally driven people sometimes feel defeated when they can't exercise, and you don't have to feel this way. I urge patients to find other coping strategies to turn to on those days when their usual exercise regimen is not an option.

Coping Strategies

Your ability to cope is like the weather in that it's different every day. Some days you may feel that you aren't coping particularly well, but don't get down on yourself. Some days are just going to suck. But having a bad day doesn't mean that you are getting worse or that you are doomed to have more bad days. Be kind to yourself on those days when you may be particularly cranky or out of it. Tomorrow you will probably feel different, and you can start again.

These are the strategies my patients often use successfully to cope with cancer and to live full lives in spite of it: distraction, optimism, gratitude, joy, meditation and prayer, humor, flow, intellectualizing, and problem solving. You may already use two or three of the following activities to help with stress. Many people have just one favorite coping strategy. But I encourage you to try several and see what works for you. It is often good to have multiple strategies.

Distraction

This is perhaps the easiest coping technique, made even easier by smartphone games, Internet surfing, and binge-watching favorite TV shows. Yes, there are times when you can—and should—distract yourself from thoughts about cancer or your symptoms and side effects. You may need distraction when waiting for test results or scans seems especially difficult or on those days when you feel more fatigued. One of my patients loves to watch the Bird Cam at Cornell Labs and also one of the many Panda Cams at various zoos, because watching animals is relaxing for her. When she can't sleep, she listens to podcasts so she can learn new things, and when she is anxious, she plays games on her smartphone. "They all tell me I'm obsessed," she says. But it's a healthy obsession, because it helps her cope. Other people spend the afternoon watching romantic comedies or classic hockey games. The point is to pass the time enjoyably while giving yourself a break.

Optimism

You can harness the power of optimism by creating some event to look forward to. Think of something that will give you pleasure, and make time to do it in the near future. This might be attending a child's or grandchild's recital, going shopping, calling a friend you haven't talked to in a while to set up a coffee date, or looking forward to watching a sporting event. You can make small plans, such as taking a day off from work to go to a matinee, or you can make big plans, such as taking a dream trip. One patient told himself that if he got through a difficult surgery, he would take his wife to Tuscany. She later said, "As soon as he got home from the hospital, he was on the Internet pricing flights and researching wines." The ability to anticipate something to look forward to—even if it's many months away—can change your whole outlook on life. Yes, there is uncertainty, so what? Just buy travel insurance.

Gratitude

In the field of positive psychology, the concept of gratitude is getting a lot of attention. Several experiments have shown that people who can write down three things for which they are grateful, and do this every day, have a better outlook on life and even have healthier relationships and life habits. Can you find and name three things for which you are grateful? You might be grateful for the companionship of a pet, a beautiful tree in your backyard, a partner who is supportive, getting your favorite infusion nurse this time, a coworker's sense of humor. On some days, finding things to name may seem difficult, but you will get better at it with practice. Ultimately, you may develop a skill that we call Velcro versus Teflon. The good things in your life will stick to you like Velcro, because you concentrate on them, while the bad things you will notice and deal with before letting them slide off of you like Teflon.

Joy

Take as many opportunities as you can to stay in the moment and enjoy simple things: a sunset, a well-played game of baseball, a good joke, a hug, a connection with a friend, nature in any form. This is something people rarely take the time to do, to really appreciate experiences as they are happening. One of my patients who lives on Cape Cod told me that she loves using her outdoor shower and now uses it all the time because it feels so good to be outside. This is using joy, doing something that feels good and enjoying every minute. Another patient told me that putting up Christmas decorations had always seemed like a chore, the first of so many to get through in an endless to-do list every December, but this year she decided that she would slow down and make hanging ornaments into an event. She also decided to go through the entire season doing only what she wanted to do, only what she knew she would enjoy.

Meditation and Prayer

Some of my patients have been meditating for many years before their cancer diagnosis, while others try it for the first time as a way of escaping the loop of worrying thoughts. People with a strong connection to a religious tradition may find prayer helpful on those days when coping seems especially difficult. Regardless of your spiritual tradition or beliefs, time for reflection is an important way to stay centered.

Humor

One of my patients likes to start his appointments by asking me whether it's still okay for him to buy green bananas. (The old jokes really are the best.) Many people have a great sense of humor and use laughter as a primary coping mechanism, and yet patients still sometimes ask whether it's okay to make jokes about having cancer. Of course it is! You have to endure a lot of craziness with cancer, and it's okay to laugh when you can and to be snarky, even edgy. No one will be offended—least of all your oncologist or your palliative care clinician. They've heard it all.

Flow

This is another concept from the field of positive psychology, and it refers to any activity that causes you to feel immersed in energized focus, involvement, and enjoyment of the process. It's different from distraction because you are doing something active and creative that is challenging without being overwhelmingly difficult. You may also think of this as being "in the zone," and some people find this feeling through work or through creative activities such as knitting, writing, or playing an instrument.

One of my patients loves painting, and she belongs to a painting club. Every two weeks, club members meet in a set location, either at the local high school or rec center, and paint together. She loves it because she can lose herself in the painting and not think of anything else. She loves the smell of the paints and the camaraderie of the fellow painters, and, even though she sometimes finds it difficult to get out of the house, she is always grateful to go to these club meetings. The idea is to find an activity that will challenge you creatively or intellectually enough to allow you to get outside yourself and to continue to grow.

Intellectualization

This is a technique you can use when you want to treat cancer the way you treat other problems, as intellectual puzzles. You may want to spend a lot of time researching all of the chemical compounds in your chemotherapy drugs and learn all about the mechanisms of how they act on cancer cells. You may want to come up with graphs and charts for side effects of treatments. You may want to research religious and spiritual texts and think about the meaning of life. These are great coping strategies that help you deal with the fact of cancer without having to think about the emotional component of your diagnosis and treatment all the time.

Problem Solving

This is a great technique on those days when you want to feel like you've accomplished something. This may mean researching alternative therapies with the plan of discussing them with your doctor. You may decide to make a financial plan to help take care of your family. You may be focused on fixing up the house, thinking, "I'm finally going to repair that cabinet door" or, "Today is the day I'm going to clean out those files." Finding practical tasks to do and problems to solve will give you a sense of control at a time when so much may seem to be out of your control.

Talking and Thinking about Difficult Topics

Part of coping is finding a way to think about and talk about difficult topics. The most important of these is the question of what you plan to do if your cancer advances or if the treatments don't work as well as you hope.

Some people are comfortable about making plans for a future in which the illness may be even more prominent in their lives, while other patients tell me that they don't want to talk about or even think about any negative possibility. They want to focus on the idea of being cured or of dealing with the cancer as a chronic illness. One patient said to me, "I don't want to think about anything other than making the cancer go away, because if I sit around worrying about dying, I'm just inviting the cancer to get worse." I had to disagree with her on several points.

First, I know that talking about a possibility doesn't make it come true. Cancer cells are driven by their own biology and not by your thoughts or anyone else's. I also know that her stated concern about wanting to think only positive thoughts was masking several other concerns that are normal and realistic. If you are dealing with a cancer diagnosis, you may be afraid that if you thoroughly consider all of the possible outcomes, you might become overwhelmed and depressed and unable to think about anything else or enjoy your life. Some people say to me, "I'm afraid that if I start crying, I may never stop." These are real concerns.

I also know that refusing to talk about your fears and about possible outcomes doesn't work very well. Think about it. It would be crazy to never have any fears or negative thoughts. So, in reality, you are not keeping the negative thoughts away; you're just sealing them off in a pressure cooker that is sure to explode later. People who try to stay stoic during the day often find that they lie awake at night or that they develop panic attacks or struggle more with fatigue. Rather than avoiding negative thoughts, you will want to find a safe way to talk about difficult topics, including your prognosis (the likely course and outcome of your disease), and what plans you may need to make if your cancer progresses. By talking about these issues and giving voice to your fears, you are taking away their power over you. It's actually easier to get back to your life after discharging your fears, if you do it in a safe way.

Opening the Box

With my patients, I often use the metaphor of the box. Everything they don't want to have to talk about or think about goes in the box. So, I ask, "Do you want to talk about your prognosis?" If the answer is no, this conversation goes in the box. "Do you want to talk about what might happen if your cancer grows through this treatment?" No? It goes in the box. We don't have to open the box until you are ready, but at some point we will have to open the box, even if it's just for a few minutes. Most patients love this idea because it gives them control over when they feel ready to talk about what may be bothering them.

I have a patient with metastatic breast cancer, and she has been in treatment for about five years. She's an intense, hard-driven person who truly believes that you can get a good outcome in anything if you work hard enough. She was initially resistant to talking about the possibility of any negative outcomes, but lately she has been wanting to open the box and have these conversations about what might happen if she can't get into a clinical trial as she hopes or what might happen if her scans show additional bone metastases. Considering all possibilities gives her the power to decide whether to get a particular surgery or radiation treatment. She can talk about how to encourage her husband to engage support services if her health gets worse. And then, when we close the box, she can go right back to talking about how she believes the right clinical trial is going to open up for her, even though she knows it's a long shot. Opening the box allows her to talk realistically about what might happen, while staying hopeful about everything else.

You can use this box idea with your doctor; you can even use it with your family. The point is to allow you and your family to stay hopeful while making room to talk about and plan for the challenges you might have to deal with, even if you don't want them to happen.

Coping with Other People

Patients sometimes tell me that the hardest challenge (emotionally) to deal with in the world of cancer is the feeling that their friends and loved ones don't know what to say and maybe even make themselves scarce for weeks or months at a time. In fact, your diagnosis may be so worrisome for other people that they either avoid the topic altogether or ask annoying and prying questions about what you are going through. In fact, there is a new line of greeting cards by Emily McDowell that captures some of this awkwardness. The message on one card reads, "I'm really sorry I haven't been in touch. I didn't know what to say." Another one says, "I promise never to try to sell you on some random treatment I read on the Internet."

It's normal to feel a little isolated at the start of treatment, while you are sorting out which of your friends and family members are going to actively support you at this time and which are going to fade into the outer circle. For some people, talking about anything that raises the idea of mortality is too much; some would rather say and do nothing than say the wrong thing while trying to help out.

Figure out whom you can rely on the most and how to manage the flow of information to extended family and friends.

The Inner and Outer Orbits

It's normal to wonder how you can talk to your friends about what's going on in your life and how to ask for the support you truly need. People often tell me that they need their friends and close family so much but don't want to overburden them. Feeling like a burden is common.

What I suggest is thinking of friends and loved ones in terms of one inner circle and several outer circles. The friends who are in your innermost orbit are the friends you know and trust the most. These are the people (and there may be just one or two) who can come to your house unannounced, ignore any clutter or mess, and, when you offer to make them coffee, cheerfully make it themselves because they already know their way around your kitchen. This is your inner orbit.

These are the people you will rely on the most, for errands, for companionship, and for commiseration. They are the ones who will never think of you as a burden. They may be terribly sad about the turn of events, but they are also the ones who can see you at your worst and roll with it. Cherish them.

Your other close friends and family—the outer orbits—may need a little help with this cancer thing, even if they love you very much. You may not feel as comfortable asking for help, and they may be less available to give it. You may have to rehearse what to say when they lower their voices and say, "How are you doing?" while looking worried. It's okay. You can come up with a pat answer to have ready, and the moment will pass. People need guidance and direction because they don't know how to say or do helpful things. The point is to speak up when you are uncomfortable. I have one patient who gets angry when family members talk about her as though she is not in the room. One of them will say, "Who is going to take Mary to the store?" And she's thinking, "I'm Mary. I'm right here. Talk to me!" She's brilliant but feels that sometimes people treat her as though she is helpless. But she's getting better at standing up for herself.

Another one of my patients was at a holiday dinner when a distant cousin turned to her and said, "Did you lose your hair everywhere?" It was an awkward moment to be sure, but at least she has a funny story to tell. The very subject of cancer is frightening to some people who have no experience with it, and they sometimes say things they immediately regret. Or maybe they regret it the next day but are too embarrassed to reach out with an apology.

Many patients learn to treat all of this with great humor. I have one patient who actually made what she called Cancer Cards. They were real cards with the word "cancer" printed on them. And when she wanted to get her way with a quarrelsome family member, she would whip out one of the cards and say, "I'm playing the cancer card." She literally trumped other people's views. Once, I think she had one of the cards with her at an amusement park, and, instead of waiting in the long line with her grandchild, she went to the front of the line and presented the card to the attendant, and said, "Excuse me, I have cancer." This was a little bit later in her illness, when she was aware of time running short. The attendant took the card, and no one objected. Sometimes it's okay to play the cancer card.

Asking for Help

Some people find it difficult to ask others to help them get along day to day because they don't want to worry anyone or feel like a burden. A patient of mine, Daniel, was in his late twenties and getting his PhD when he was diagnosed with sarcoma. Initially he was deeply conflicted about having anyone help him. He believed that he needed to maintain his independence and do everything for himself. He thought it would help his family feel more confident about how he was coping if he told them he didn't need any help after infusions. In truth, they just became more worried. They called constantly asking whether he needed any help and offering to shop and cook for him. His parents were beside themselves imagining that he was feeling awful in his apartment by himself.

After several tense exchanges with his family, Daniel realized he needed a different approach. He made a list of everything that would make his life easier if someone could help, including laundry, grocery shopping, being with him to get back and forth to the bathroom those first couple days after chemo. He told me he realized that his friends and family couldn't go through the cancer treatment but he could let them be connected with him by letting them help. He told me, "The best way I can love them is by letting them help me. It just took me a while to figure that one out."

Extended Family and Community

Those closest to you will be in contact with you every day and may even come to appointments with you. But what about everybody else? If you have a large extended family or a large social network, you may want to have someone send a group e-mail with some basic facts about your diagnosis and what kind of help would be appreciated. I know of one rabbi who did this. He sent out a group e-mail to the members of his temple to inform them that his wife had received a cancer diagnosis. What was great about this letter is that it reassured his congregation that his wife was getting excellent care and didn't have any immediate needs. It was also clear about what the couple did and didn't want in terms of communication. It stated that while they welcomed good thoughts and prayers, they didn't want to receive phone calls or e-mails in the near term. The couple felt an obligation to be honest with members, but they also knew that the last thing they needed was an endlessly ringing phone so that people could say some version of "I'm sorry." If you are going to send out a group e-mail, it's important to state what you do and don't want from the people receiving it.

The letter also directed recipients to a website where a temple member was coordinating efforts to help the couple. There are several websites that do this. One of them is called Care Calendar, and another is called Lotsa Helping Hands. These websites become a clearinghouse for coordinating all kinds of help, including prepared meals, visits from friends, dog walking, or rides to medical appointments. These kinds of websites give people concrete ways to offer help, which makes them feel so much better than offering the vague, "Let me know if I can do anything."

Some people start a blog to keep everyone informed of what they are going through and what they are thinking along the way. What's great about this is that you can include as much or as little information as you like. Even if you don't use a website or blog, you can assign someone to serve as the communications czar, the person who will get medical updates to extended family and who will field questions people may not be comfortable asking directly. This person can also set up a schedule for others who want to help with visits or giving the kids rides to school. This can make a big difference for you and give people an opportunity to support you in ways that you need.

8

How Do I Cope with Changes in My Body?

PATIENTS OFTEN TELL ME THAT the physical changes brought about by cancer treatment are the most challenging to deal with. "My body is so different," they say to me. "I don't recognize myself anymore." People with cancer may experience noticeable weight loss or hair loss or surgery that alters their bodies. It's tough to look at yourself in the bathroom mirror and see scars or a face swollen from steroids, or to walk differently because of neuropathy. A big part of living well with cancer is figuring out who you are in this new body and how you relate to others even though you may be wondering whether they look at you differently and whether they see you as a cancer patient rather than a person.

It's hard to know which changes are going to be the most difficult for you. I saw a woman at the clinic recently who had been living with breast cancer for more than five years. Julie had gone through a mastectomy and several cycles of chemotherapy in which she had lost a significant amount of weight. And yet she prided herself on not letting the diagnosis define her. She continued to work nearly full time, and she still went to the gym several times per week. Now, for the first time, she was losing her hair as a result of treatment. Julie told me how strange it was to look at herself in the mirror with her new wig. "I feel like a cancer patient now," Julie said to me. "I haven't until this point." For her, the idea that acquaintances and strangers would look at her differently was the hardest part. She worried that wearing a wig was like wearing a sign that says, "I have cancer." And she worried that people would want her to talk about her diagnosis even when she didn't feel like talking about it.

In this chapter, I'll describe some ways to cope with these physical changes that can be temporary, such as hair loss, or that are permanent, such as ostomy bags. And I'll talk about changes in intimate relationships and sexual function and how to cope with those.

Hair Loss

Losing your hair is hard for everyone, but especially for women who live with a cultural expectation of having not just hair but a hairstyle. I advise people to ask the oncology team about the likelihood that any regimen will result in hair loss and when it might occur. Oncologists and oncology nurses know how different regimens often affect patients. Still, they may not always be accurate, as everyone reacts differently. Julie had told me that her oncologist estimated that just 5 percent of people lose their hair on her regimen, and she turned out to be in that minority. So she was happy that she had gone to a wig store to get a high-quality wig made before she lost her hair. The fitter was able to see how she wore her hair while she had it and crafted a wig that was in keeping with that style. Wigs can be expensive, depending on the type that you choose, and many insurers don't cover this cost. Also, wigs made of 100 percent human hair often need more upkeep than those made of other materials. Some people ultimately don't like wearing a wig and opt for scarves or hats instead.

There is a lot of advice online about how to manage the actual hair loss as it's happening. Sometimes hair loss is gradual and sometimes rapid, and you may see advice to keep your hair close cropped or to shave your head as the thinning progresses to keep from dealing with hair coming out in clumps. After you experience hair loss, you may notice that you get cold more easily and that the skin on your scalp is more sensitive and more vulnerable to sunburn.

For many people, the best part of chemotherapy-induced hair loss is that their hair will grow back when the treatment regimen ends or changes. Hair should start to regrow about three weeks after your last treatment. Julie's concerns about wearing a wig eased when she realized that some coworkers didn't notice it, and those who may have noticed knew better than to comment.

Neuropathy

Some patients experience pronounced neuropathy during chemo-therapy. They may have numbness or pain in their hands that inter-feres with writing and typing or fastening buttons. Some people have decreased sensation in their feet, affecting the way they walk. They may have to step carefully. I've had patients say that their grand-kids ask them why they suddenly seem so frail. And they feel frail, as though their bodies don't work as well as they should. Avid golfers have trouble setting up shots or walking through a golf course because they have lost a strong sense of balance. I had a patient who used to go to the local Y to work out every day, was part of a biking team, and was a serious runner who competed in multiple races a year but now has to confine himself to swimming laps, because it's safer to be in a pool than to be out running or biking. Dave usually tells patients that it can take months for neuropathy to heal, and sometimes you won't feel normal again for up to a year. But when you stop using the chemotherapy regimen that is causing the nerve problems, most neuropathies will resolve over time. However, some neuropathies get better but never completely go away.

Getting Used to a New Body

My patients have gone through mastectomies, or they have had G-tubes, or gastric (feeding) tubes, inserted. They live with ostomies that help drain fluids, or they have fluid buildup in the abdomen. In some cases, they take steroids or other medication that causes facial swelling, or they have bowel changes that mean they have to be near a bathroom much of the time. All of these changes make patients feel that they have exchanged their familiar body for something else, and it takes time to get used to this new body. I remind patients that there is a loss related to these changes, and it's absolutely normal to grieve these losses.

It's also important to figure out who you are in this new body, and make strategies for how to live with these changes. This may mean asking questions about physical changes even before you have significant surgeries. A patient of mine who was about to get a G-tube for supplemental nutrition asked me, "Can I swim with one of those?" Swimming was one of Margaret's favorite activities, and she didn't want to give up swimming with her grandchildren in the summer. I didn't know, but with a little research I found that the answer is yes. For Margaret, the ability to focus on what she could do that gave her joy helped her go through the surgery that would change the way she eats. Even if these changes have already occurred, you can think about the activities you love to do and can still do in this new body. You can find a new normal.

Some people put energy into looking as normal as possible because that gives them more confidence as they continue to work and socialize. My patient Tara had metastatic ovarian cancer (it had spread beyond the ovaries). Over time she needed both a tube for draining fluid from her abdomen and kidney tubes to drain urine. It was essential to Tara to maintain her sense of fashion despite these bulky encumbrances. She found some stylish pants with an elastic waistband and paired those with flowing scarves that she knotted over her shoulders. When she lost her hair, she wore a wig until summer, when she gave it up in favor of a straw hat. She told me, "I just needed to figure out my new style."

Many people feel alone at first in these changes because they have never known anyone who had to deal with these issues. But you aren't alone. There are lots of people going through the same challenges; many of them have written blogs about the experience or have created websites that detail great coping strategies. Some have even designed products to help others like themselves. By reading some of these accounts, you may find that these physical changes don't need to define you. They are simply part of the new you.

These body changes also may be unsettling for your partner. Remember that your partner may be grieving the loss of changes in your body. The sooner you both can become comfortable with this new body, the better.

Changes in Sexuality

My patients are sometimes reluctant to talk about how their cancer affects intimacy with their partner. Patients may have strong feelings about their new bodies that make it difficult to feel attractive or sexy. One of my patients who had a double mastectomy told me that it took her several months after her physical recovery before she felt like having sex again. "My husband told me that I was beautiful and I believed him. And he told me that he didn't marry me for my breasts. I knew he was okay with it. I just needed some time to feel beautiful again in this new body, but it happened."

Cancer treatment can also change sexual function. It can affect sexual organs, functioning, and drive. Sometimes factors related to the illness like pain or fatigue make actually having sex too tough. You don't have to assume that intercourse will be difficult forever, but it may be difficult right now. And I also remind people that sexual intercourse is just one way to be intimate with your partner.

Intimacy and Sex

Some couples feel that they ought to be having sex, even when intercourse has become tricky because of cancer treatment. Sometimes the patient with cancer feels a sense of obligation to his or her partner, or in some cases, people think that having sex would make them feel more like themselves. Partners sometimes also want to initiate sex, because they want to reaffirm the intimacy that they feel or because they want their partner to feel more whole and to feel loved and appreciated. Couples need to talk about these issues and see whether each person wants the same things. It's easy for couples to make assumptions about what the other person wants or needs emotionally and physically.

Cancer and treatment can affect your ability to have sex in the way you have before. Your doctor may not raise the issue of sexuality and sexual function, but continuing to be intimate with your partner is a meaningful part of living fully with cancer. Raising these issues with your medical team is part of advocating for yourself and your needs. Many large cancer centers have sexual health clinics and specialists who can help patients deal with the ways in which cancer has affected their sexuality.

I like to remind couples that intimacy isn't the same thing as having intercourse. They know this already, but it's good for people who have been coupled for a long time to remember that intimacy comes from all kinds of touching. Intercourse can give way to caressing, holding, hugging, and kissing. Holding your partner's hand is not the same as holding the hand of your child or your friend. You can maintain tremendous intimacy with your partner, even if you can't have sex in the way that you have in the past. The idea of intimacy can change and become much more emotional.

Sexual health specialists will also say that intimacy is sometimes a loaded word. It sounds like serious work, and in reality sex is a form of play. You can and should playfully explore the body that you have now, focusing on sensations. What feels good? Erogenous zones can change after cancer treatment, but they are still there. If intercourse is stressful, you can always step back to what feels good.

Logistics of Intercourse

Many patients and their partners feel daunted by the logistics of sex. They have so many questions: Is it safe? Can my partner get exposed to the chemotherapy? Is there risk of infection? What if I get pregnant? What if it hurts?

Is it safe? While the risk of passing chemotherapy to a partner is probably very small and largely unknown, most doctors will tell you to use a condom during the first two weeks after an infusion.

Risk of infection. There are times after an infusion when you are at higher risk of developing an infection, and your team may advise against sexual intercourse during this time, usually seven to ten days after an infusion, when your white count is at its lowest point. Also, if your oncology team is worried about your risk of infection because you have a low white blood cell count, you will want to use condoms to minimize your exposure to sexually transmitted diseases.

Risk of pregnancy. Getting pregnant on most disease-modifying therapy would not be safe. You need to ask your medical team whether this is the case for you. Every regimen is different.

Pain management. Some partners worry that they will hurt the patient during sex. If pain has been an issue in treatment, you will want to use proactive pain management. Work with your team to make sure your pain is well controlled. You may also need to pre-medicate with a breakthrough pain medication (see chapter 11) one hour before sex to ensure more comfort. I also remind people to think about different positions and ways of pleasuring yourself and your partner if intercourse is too painful. Sometimes side positions are easier and require less energy. But you might also consider alternative forms of sexual intimacy to penetration.

Fatigue. This is another common barrier to having sex and may require some planning to work around it, because there aren't many treatments for fatigue. Most people with cancer-related fatigue do say there is a time of day when they feel most energetic. That would be a time to think about initiating sex. I also remind patients that fatigue gets worse when you have other symptoms that aren't controlled, so work with your medical team to treat them.

Working around ostomies and tubes. Some people feel self-conscious about having sex when they have an ostomy bag or other external tube. Many couples work around this by trying different positions. I had one patient with an ostomy bag after her colon cancer surgery, and her solution was to wear a beautiful silk camisole over it. Her husband didn't mind the bag at all, but the camouflage helped her to feel sexy.

Physical Issues with Intercourse

Cancer treatment can also change your ability to engage in intercourse. For men, some cancer treatments change their ability to obtain and maintain an erection. Erectile function requires an intact nervous system in the lumbosacral (lower) spine and pelvis as well as an intact vascular system in the pelvis. Both of these can be affected by age or by medical conditions such as diabetes. (In fact, erectile dysfunction is common among men who are long-term diabetics.) Surgery and radiation administered to the pelvis can affect both the vascular system and nervous system and contribute to erectile dysfunction. If this happens, patients can take a class of drugs called phosphodiesterase inhibitors, such as sildenafil (Viagra) that can help with the vascular system and make it easier to get or maintain an erection.

However, if the nervous system has been disabled in the pelvis or lower spine, these drugs might not have any effect. I usually tell men that the only way to find out is to try them and see whether they work. If they don't, men can work with a urologist to explore other options, such as penile implants.

Libido and erectile function are also sensitive to the levels of testosterone that a man produces. Both chemotherapy and radiation treatments in the pelvis can cause low testosterone, and it's important to check this level when you want to know what's causing erectile dysfunction. There are testosterone replacement therapies that men can take, but some cancers such as prostate cancer are sensitive to testosterone. You don't want to take any hormone therapies that will make your cancer worse, so ask your oncologist if it's okay to take a testosterone replacement.

Women can also have difficulties with intercourse during and after treatment. Postmenopausal women and those who have been made menopausal by chemotherapy, radiation, or surgery can experience vaginal dryness. Some treatments for vaginal dryness include vitamin E suppositories or over-the-counter lubricants. There are also estrogen creams that can really help. You will want to ask your oncologist about the safety of using products that contain estrogen if you have a hormone-sensitive cancer, such as breast cancer. Some oncologists won't want you to use any product that contains any estrogen if you have a cancer that is sensitive to hormones in your body. The safest lubricants are water based and don't contain any oils or hormonal supplements.

Women who have had radiation treatments to the pelvis sometimes experience scarring of the vagina that makes intercourse difficult or impossible. You should talk to your oncologist about the risk of this happening as you start radiation treatments. Vaginal dilators that doctors can use during radiation treatments can help prevent this scarring and preserve a woman's ability to have intercourse after the radiation therapy ends.

The bottom line is that you should feel free to be open about all sexual issues with your treatment team. Some hospitals and practices have started dedicated sexual dysfunction clinics or have physicians who are known for their expertise in this area. Most oncologists can handle the basic questions and issues, but a dedicated specialist is often needed to answer more complex questions and issues. So ask your treatment team where you can get help for any sexual dysfunction.

PART II

Managing Symptoms and Side Effects

9

Controlling Nausea

EVERYONE ASSOCIATES CHEMOTHERAPY TREATMENTS WITH nausea. But there are many triggers for nausea or vomiting while you are a cancer patient. It might seem that nausea is pretty simple. Something is wrong and you feel crummy. Or you feel crummy and you are throwing up. It's awful and you just want someone to do something.

Medically, nausea is complicated because it can be triggered by the brain, by the stomach and intestines, by infection, by the medications you are taking, and even by your mood. Each of these causes has a different set of techniques to solve the problem. Doctors have to consider a lot of factors when treating nausea, and one of my colleagues came up with a mnemonic (VOMITING) to help us remember all of them. This may sound a little nerdy, but what can you do? When your doctor starts asking a lot of questions about your nausea, you'll know that he or she is thinking along these lines:

V = Vestibular, anything happening in the brain or inner ear that makes you dizzy.
O = Obstruction, meaning anything in the stomach or colon that may be blocking food from digesting. This includes constipation.

M = Motility, meaning the stomach and intestines aren't pushing food along, and it's sitting in your system.

I = Infection or inflammation that can be in the stomach or intestines or even in your throat.

T = Toxins, which means any medications you are taking can cause the side effect of nausea, such as chemotherapy or opioids for pain.

I = Intracranial process, which means nausea can be caused by brain metastases (tumors that have moved from their original location to the brain) or an infection that affects the brain or spinal cord.

N = Nerves, meaning anxiety or anticipatory nausea.

G = Gums and oropharynx, meaning that mouth sores, dry mouth, or a yeast infection in your mouth can affect your ability or willingness to eat.

What Your Doctor Will Ask You

When you call or come to the clinic and talk about nausea or being unable to eat, your medical team will ask numerous questions to determine the cause. If you can give your medical team answers, you will help them find a cause and a solution:

- Do you feel nausea all the time?
- Does eating make the feeling better or worse?
- Is the nausea worse with certain foods? Or after taking certain pills?
- Are you vomiting?
- When you vomit, is it food you ate a while ago? Or is it just bile?
- Do you have any acid reflux symptoms?
- Are you moving your bowels regularly?
- Do you feel constipated?
- Are you having headaches?
- Have you been able to eat and drink?
- Are you having abdominal pain associated with vomiting?

Common Sources of Nausea

There are several general categories of causes of nausea. I will describe each one, starting with the most common, and describe the way your doctor may treat it.

Medications That Cause Nausea

When you tell your doctor about nausea, the first thing he or she will think about is that your medications or treatment may be the culprit. Almost any medication can cause nausea, but, for cancer patients, we know that the most common sources are the chemotherapy itself and the opioids used to treat pain.

Chemotherapy-Induced Nausea

Of course, everyone knows that chemotherapy can cause nausea. Not all of these drugs have this side effect, but many of them do. We have great medications that reduce or eliminate nausea after infusions. The process of vomiting is called emesis, and the drugs that prevent nausea and vomiting are referred to as antiemetics. In general, five classes of antiemetics are commonly used to treat nausea caused by chemotherapy (table 9.1). Occasionally we have to go beyond these classes of drugs to control nausea, but thankfully that's a rare event.

Chemotherapy drugs are classified into one of three categories based on their tendency to cause nausea: low emetogenic potential, moderate emetogenic potential, and high emetogenic potential. Depending on the emetogenic potential of the chemotherapy you are on, your doctor will prescribe the appropriate drug or mix of drugs to prevent nausea. Each type of antiemetic uses different mechanisms to prevent nausea, which is why it is safe to use more than one drug at the same time if the doctor thinks that nausea could be a problem on your regimen. Oncologists almost never use two drugs from the same category because they will have overlapping side effects.

For people getting chemotherapy regimens with low emetogenic potential, doctors might not prescribe an antinausea drug.

TABLE 9.1 *Five classes of antiemetics*

Class	Commonly used medications
Steroids	Dexamethasone (Decadron)
Benzodiazepines	Lorazepam (Ativan)
Dopamine receptor antagonists	Prochlorperazine (Compazine)
	Metoclopramide (Reglan)
5HT3 or serotonin antagonists	Ondansetron (Zofran)
	Granisetron (Kytril)
	Palonosetron (Aloxi)
NK1 receptor antagonists	Aprepitant (Emend)
	Fosaprepitant (Emend for injection)

5HT3 Antagonists

Most intravenous chemotherapy regimens fall into the moderately emetogenic category, and the most common method used to treat this class of nausea is a combination of 5HT3 antagonists and steroids. Patients take these 5HT3 antagonists such as ondansetron (Zofran) and palonosetron (Aloxi) prior to getting chemotherapy. Palonosetron actually acts for three more days, and you won't need to give yourself any additional doses of this medication. But ondansetron will work for only eight hours at standard doses. If your doctor prescribes ondansetron, you will be instructed to take this medication every eight hours for three days after your infusion. It's important to ask your infusion nurse which 5HT3 antagonist you are receiving and whether you will need to take more of it in the coming days.

There are pros and cons to each of the different types of 5HT3 antagonists. For most people, these drugs manage the nausea effectively. You may not feel much like eating during this time, but you shouldn't feel actively sick.

The primary side effect of 5HT3 antagonists is constipation, which occurs in about a third of patients who take them. Your doctor may suggest a laxative for you to take if this happens. The reason to treat constipation even if you aren't eating much is that constipation can also cause nausea.

Steroids Used with 5HT3 Antagonists

The 5HT3 antagonists often work better when they are given with a steroid, and the most commonly used steroid is dexamethasone. Steroids are safe to take in short episodes, but they can also cause uncomfortable side effects. The most common steroid side effect is a sudden, short burst of energy that lasts for two or three days. People often have trouble sleeping and can be incredibly energetic and creative. I've had husbands and wives complain to me that their spouse is up all night on some type of house project that keeps everyone awake. Then when the effect wears off they can crash and sleep for hours on end. The other major side effect of steroids is that they can make your blood glucose run high. If you are diabetic or have a tendency toward high blood sugar, your oncology team may want to monitor your blood sugar levels and may even need to adjust your diabetes medications while you are taking dexamethasone.

You may be wondering why we start with these two medications if they can cause all of these side effects. The problem with nausea and vomiting is that once it starts it can be very hard to get under control again with medications. Also, most people fear nausea so much when they start chemotherapy that doctors want to keep this side effect under control from the beginning. Many doctors start by prescribing high doses of antinausea medication to make sure that the first chemotherapy cycle goes as smoothly as possible. If it goes well, your doctor will probably pare down the medication in subsequent cycles until you find the dose that controls nausea with a minimum of side effects.

NK-1 Antagonists

If you are on a chemotherapy regimen that has a high potential to cause nausea, your doctor might prescribe NK-1 antagonists in addition to steroids and 5HT3 antagonists. These drugs can be dramatically effective. So if you experience severe nausea despite taking 5HT3 antagonists and steroids, don't despair. We've had many patients successfully control nausea when we add one of these medications.

For example, I had a sixty-three-year-old patient, Ada, with stomach cancer who was referred to palliative care after her third round of treatment, in part because she was losing a lot of weight. I asked her how chemotherapy was going and she said fine, but her daughters looked pretty angry. I asked whether she had any nausea, and she said that she had no nausea during the first two days, and then she held herself very still. At this point, one of her daughters interrupted to say that Ada had been really sick during the third and fourth days after infusion. "It was horrible," said the daughter. After some more questioning, I found that Ada had heard the doctor tell her that her nausea would be worst during the first two days and then should get better because that's how it is for most patients. So, Ada had stopped taking her antiemetics forty-eight hours after each infusion, only to feel sick and unable to keep anything down for the next two days. She had gone through this three times without saying anything to her oncologist, and she had begun to dread infusions to the point where she couldn't eat much on the day before.

While it's important to listen to the oncologist and the infusion nurses, who are excellent sources of information about side effects, it's even more important to listen to your body. I tell people to keep a record of their symptoms after the first infusion, how much they ate and drank and how they felt. This is important information to give to the nurses and doctors, who can adjust your medications to make the next infusion easier. Your body is different from everyone else's, and you may react differently to treatment. The point is that you should never feel that you should expect nausea and have to suffer through it. You don't have to feel sick. If you feel nausea after an infusion, contact the clinic right away and tell them how this is affecting your life, because your oncology team or your palliative care clinician can and should prescribe something else to help you.

In Ada's case, I knew that the first thing she needed was to take the antiemetics for at least another day, maybe two. If that failed to control her nausea, I would add aprepitant (Emend), one of the NK-1 antagonists. I was fairly certain that we could get her to a better place, and sure enough she was doing markedly better after the next cycle of chemotherapy.

Benzodiazepines for Nausea

A few patients have nausea even with all of these precautions, and we call this breakthrough nausea, because it breaks through the antiemetics. Don't give up if you experience some breakthrough nausea. Your doctor can still prescribe something to help. In this case, you might be given prochlorperazine (Compazine) or lorazepam (Ativan) for additional help. These other two classes of agents, dopamine receptor antagonists and benzodiazepines, are typically used for the occasional breakthrough nausea.

They can be particularly effective in specific circumstances. For instance, lorazepam is a great drug for anticipatory nausea, which is a type of nausea that some people feel when they are just walking into the hospital or infusion unit. It's possible that the mere thought of getting the chemotherapy or the smell of a hospital will make a few people nauseated. Benzodiazepines are also very effective at preventing this type of nausea.

The other benefit of lorazepam is that you don't have to swallow it. Instead, you can let it melt under your tongue. Sometimes, I get calls at night from patients whose antinausea medication has worn off. Their nausea prevents them from swallowing any pills to help. I tell them to put a lorazepam tablet under their tongue and let it melt. In fifteen minutes, they feel well enough to swallow their other antinausea medications.

Staying Ahead of Chemo-Induced Nausea

Many times, patients think they should take these medications only after they start to feel crummy, but you need to be taking them around the clock for the first three days to get the full benefit. Other patients stop taking them too soon, and then they start to feel sick, at which point the medication needs time to take effect. It's much easier to stay ahead of nausea than to play catch-up once the nausea starts. That's why doctors are often insistent that patients take medications to prevent nausea even if they aren't feeling sick.

You should expect that any chemo-induced nausea will be well controlled. Here's what you can do to help:

- Take your antiemetics exactly as prescribed.
- If your team has given a regimen that needs to be taken around the clock, do it. Don't wait for the nausea to start. The goal is to prevent the nausea from coming on.
- Tell your team if the regimen they prescribed is not working. There are other options.
- Don't let yourself get dehydrated. Keep drinking water, even if you don't feel like eating.
- If you are having real trouble keeping fluids down, you might need to get some IV fluid.
- If your team is having a tough time managing the nausea, ask for a palliative care consult.

Opioid-Induced Nausea

Opioids are the medications your doctor may prescribe to help with pain. They do a great job of controlling pain, but they have the unfortunate side effect of causing nausea in two different ways. They can directly affect parts of your brain responsible for nausea, such as the chemoreceptor trigger zone and the vomiting center. They also can cause your digestion to slow down, which results in constipation that can eventually lead to nausea. Some people experience nausea in the first few days of starting the medication. For most patients the nausea goes away after those first three to five days. We just need to treat the nausea with effective medications until the body gets used to the pain medication. Dopamine antagonists such as prochlorperazine (Compazine) can be quite effective. We suggest patients take them every six to eight hours for those first few days. Some patients react differently to different opioids. So for example, morphine may cause nausea in one person but not in another, and the same is true for oxycodone, hydromorphone, and fentanyl.

In most cases, your body gets used to pain medication, and the nausea goes away after the first few days. Talk to your doctor about the possibility that pain medication may be causing your nausea. You might have to take a lower dose at first.

Also remember to take laxatives to treat the constipation caused by the opioids, even after the first few days. The constipation side effect of opioids does not go away. As long as you are on opioids, you will probably need to take laxatives (what doctors sometimes call a "bowel regimen") every day.

Obstructions That Cause Nausea

Nausea can also result from some kind of mechanical problem or obstruction in the gastrointestinal (GI) tract. All of your digestion takes place in what is essentially a long tube that runs from your mouth through the esophagus, stomach, intestines, and to the rectum. Your body moves food along through a series of involuntary muscle contractions, so nutrients and waste are pushed from one section of the GI tract to the next. Any number of factors can interfere with this process and back up the system, which can cause nausea.

Gastroparesis

This is one of the most common causes of nausea, particularly when the nausea is constant. It's a technical term that means your stomach isn't emptying of food. Everything you have eaten is sort of sitting there because the stomach isn't contracting enough to move it into the intestines. After a while, your stomach signals the nausea centers in your brain. There are several reasons this may be happening. Sometimes pain medications, such as opioids, dull the activity in the GI tract. Sometimes you might have severe constipation, and if the intestines can't empty, the stomach can't either. Perhaps there is a tumor in the intestines or stomach that is interfering with digestion. You can suspect gastroparesis if your nausea is pretty much constant and if you are vomiting food you have eaten hours before.

Your doctor will be looking for an underlying cause of this nausea, but the ultimate goal is to get the food moving again so that you feel better. There are several medications that can help, including metoclopramide (Reglan) or erythromycin, which is an antibiotic that has the side effect of kicking the digestive tract into high gear.

Whenever you have gastroparesis, your doctor is going to ask about your bowel movements as well, because he or she wants to make sure to treat any underlying constipation that may be contributing to your stomach troubles as well.

Constipation

This is the most common cause of nausea after chemotherapy-induced nausea. If you've been in treatment any length of time and have been taking antinausea medications or opioids for pain, you know about constipation (see chapter 10). If your constipation is bad enough to cause general nausea, you probably need to adjust your dose of laxatives or the frequency with which you take them. Don't be afraid to bring this up with your doctor. Helping you get this under control should be a priority for your medical team. Some patients choose to reduce the antinausea medications they take after a chemotherapy infusion because they would rather endure short-term nausea than deal with constipation that makes them feel crummy later. This is a trade-off that you can make as a patient.

Upper Airway Irritation

Sometimes patients will have gagging or coughing that can cause vomiting with or without any real nausea. This can be caused by thick oral or nasal secretions that trigger gagging. Sometimes you can start coughing and then eventually the cough triggers a gag reflex even though you aren't feeling sick. I had a patient with lung cancer who developed pneumonia that caused severe coughing. Sure enough, she would start a coughing jag, and it would end with her vomiting what she ate.

Sometimes the cause is harder to pinpoint. One of Dave's patients who had hepatocellular cancer, a common form of liver cancer, also struggled with nausea. Dave kept changing his medications to try to get on top of it, but nothing seemed to work. Then the patient mentioned that he had a cottony substance in his mouth. Dave took a look and saw immediately that the patient had a yeast infection in his mouth, likely exacerbated by the steroids he needed to take with his chemotherapy regimen. An upper endoscopy revealed that his esophagus was coated by the infection, which no doubt caused nausea.

After two days of antifungal treatments, the yeast infection subsided and the nausea disappeared as well.

In these situations, keep talking to your doctor about anything that seems related to your nausea. We want to treat the cough or find the underlying irritation.

Abdominal Tumors

As cancer progresses, you can develop tumors either in the lining of the abdomen, called peritoneal carcinomatosis, or inside the bowels.

The peritoneum is a thin membrane that covers the organs in the abdomen. Sometimes a tumor will metastasize to the membrane and cause the bowels to function erratically. It can look like a spider web growing over the intestines making it difficult for them to move effectively, which causes nausea and bloating. The best treatment for this is treating the cancer itself. It's also very important to have any underlying constipation under control because constipation will make the symptoms from peritoneal carcinomatosis worse.

You can also develop a tumor inside the small bowel or stomach that can cause nausea along with severe abdominal pain. In this case, the nausea won't improve even if you take antiemetics. You also have to be careful when taking medications such as metoclopramide (see table 9.1) when your doctor is worried about a complete obstruction. This class of medications can make the intestines push harder against an obstruction that's not going to move. Ultimately, that will cause more pain and you risk causing a tear in the bowels, which is dangerous.

Liver Dysfunction

The liver's job is to rid the body of toxins. If the liver is having trouble functioning, these toxins may build up and cause nausea. Also, if you have tumors growing in the liver, they can affect the way the stomach pushes food through to the intestines, meaning that liver tumors can contribute to gastroparesis. If it's not possible to treat the underlying cause of liver dysfunction, you can ask your doctor about the possibility of taking antinausea medications. Remember that you may need to take them at a lower dose than normal if your liver is having trouble metabolizing medications.

Neurologic Causes of Nausea

Your brain contains receptors that help coordinate and initiate the act of vomiting. This is a safety measure that helps the body rid the stomach of toxins. So you can imagine that anything that affects your brain or the vestibular nerve (which regulates balance) can cause you to feel or be sick. A metastasis in your brain can cause swelling that increases the pressure in these nausea centers and makes you feel sick. If this is the case, you will probably—but not always—experience a headache as well. If you have nausea along with a headache, you need to alert your oncology team. Often doctors will prescribe steroids to decrease the swelling in the brain. You may also need radiation or surgery to treat the tumors.

Sensory Causes of Nausea

All different kinds of sensory inputs can induce nausea. Some of my patients will be doing fine and then smell something that triggers an intense reaction. It might be the smell or sight of food, even foods they had previously loved. Chemotherapy can cause short-term nausea after an infusion, but it can also cause a low-grade nausea that is sensitive to strong smells. It's sort of like being pregnant and having a reaction to certain kinds of smells. Remember that this won't last forever.

I had a patient who loved his family's pasta sauce and the Sunday night ritual of having the family over for dinner. While he was in chemotherapy, he couldn't eat it at all. Even the smell of the sauce cooking made him sick, which was upsetting both for him and for his family. He felt like he wasn't himself anymore and that he couldn't enjoy the simplest pleasure of eating his favorite food. But then when he switched to a new line of chemotherapy, the feeling went away and he could dig in just like he could before. So you may need to avoid certain foods while you are in a certain chemotherapy regimen and look for foods that are more appealing. Trust your body and be kind to yourself while you are getting through this time. You may want to drink smoothies or protein supplement drinks if you need to. Many people find that eating smaller meals more frequently can be a good strategy. You may find that you need really small portions at first. A whole muffin might be overwhelming, so start with a half or a quarter and work your way up.

Anxiety

You may have had a feeling of anxiety that was so intense that you actually felt sick to your stomach. That's because anxiety can cause nausea, and if you are feeling anxious during treatment or if you are having trouble with issues not related to treatment, these feelings can create or exacerbate nausea.

If you don't want to take antianxiety medications to treat the anxiety, you can look into cognitive behavioral therapy (a form of psychotherapy in which the patient works with a therapist on the interaction of thoughts and behaviors on feelings; see chapter 12) and get some techniques for calming down during stressful times. But anxiety can also be treated effectively with a low dose of lorazepam (Ativan) or olanzapine (Zyprexa). Lorazepam can cause confusion in some people, and in that case olanzapine can be a better choice.

Nausea is a blanket term that covers a lot of possible causes, and treating nausea requires ongoing interaction with your medical team. It's important to tell the clinicians about your nausea whenever it occurs. This is one of those symptoms, like pain, in which you need to be proactive with your medical team because they have tools to help you and they want you to feel your best.

10

Managing Constipation, Diarrhea, and Bowel Obstruction

BOWEL MOVEMENTS ARE A POPULAR subject with oncologists. It's sad but true that you are going to be called upon to describe them at virtually every appointment. This is because cancer can directly affect your bowels, making you constipated, while chemotherapy often causes diarrhea. On top of this, many of the medications we prescribe to treat nausea and pain can cause constipation. You will likely experience both constipation and diarrhea during the course of treatment, and your medical team will need to have near-constant dialog with you about changes in your bowel function as a result. Don't worry. Your doctor has a lot of strategies to use to treat both of these conditions and help you feel more comfortable. If you are seriously struggling, your doctor may order scans to see what may be causing you trouble. This chapter will cover constipation caused by either treatment or the cancer itself, and what your team will do to treat this. It will also talk about treatments for diarrhea caused by chemotherapy or infection.

How the GI Tract Works

Doctors take the unromantic view of the GI tract as a long hose that handles intake at the mouth and esophagus, processes nutrition in the stomach and small intestine, and eliminates waste through the colon, rectum, and anus (figure 10.1). We also think of the movement of food, nutrition, and waste as a transit system. This transit is managed by muscular contractions in the wall of the GI tract called peristalsis. You may know and be able to feel how the esophagus pushes food down into your stomach; the stomach and intestines also push food along with similar contractions. So does the colon and rectum.

Peristalsis is governed by a complex system of nerves that are autonomic, meaning that you don't have any voluntary control over them. Doctors are only beginning to understand this GI nervous system—sometimes called the enteric nervous system—and all the ways in which it works to regulate digestion and even hunger. We do know that it is connected through a series of hormones to the central nervous system. It consists of about five hundred million neurons, many more than you have in your spinal cord.

There are numerous ways that cancer and cancer treatment can affect the enteric nervous system and the body's ability to regulate digestion. Many chemotherapy regimens affect the cells lining the intestines and increase transit time in the bowels, which leads to diarrhea. Other medications that treat pain and chemo-induced nausea often have the side effect of slowing down peristalsis throughout the GI tract or in the lower bowels specifically. This can cause sudden and severe constipation.

People sometimes think that they can regulate their bowels through diet alone. Diet does matter, and foods such as chocolate and pizza can be very constipating, while diets rich in fiber from grains and salads can increase the rate at which stool goes through the GI tract. So if you have constipation or diarrhea caused by treatment or medication, certain dietary choices can make the situation worse.

The problem is that medications can have powerful effects on how your bowels function, and it's almost impossible to counteract these effects through diet alone.

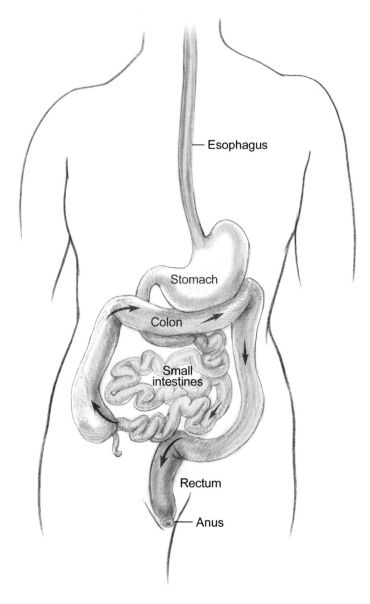

Figure 10.1 The gastrointestinal tract

Cycling between Constipation and Diarrhea

Regulating your bowels during chemotherapy treatment is tricky. Most people taking antiemetics, or antinausea drugs, will have constipation for the first week after an infusion. Then in the second week, when they have stopped taking the antiemetics, they may experience diarrhea from the chemotherapy itself. People in chemotherapy often toggle between constipation and diarrhea, and this can be very frustrating. Figuring out a short course of laxatives takes time.

I always tell my patients that we probably can't make it perfect, but we can make the situation livable. Treating constipation is often more art than science, and it may take several infusions for your medical team to get a handle on things.

I also ask patients to tell me which side effect they fear more, the constipation or the diarrhea. Most people who have experienced both say that they don't like diarrhea, but that they truly hate constipation. I get it. When you are constipated, you often feel uncomfortable. Many people don't feel like doing anything and they don't feel social. By contrast, while diarrhea is never pleasant, it isn't painful, and most people can function pretty well between episodes.

Signs of Constipation

Everyone who has experienced constipation knows the telltale signs of feeling bloated, maybe feeling discomfort in the bowels or cramping in the lower left quadrant of the abdomen. Even if you don't feel these symptoms, you may want to be aware of some other signs of constipation and bring them up with your medical team:

- Not moving your bowels every day or every other day, if you did so before starting cancer treatment.
- Failing to move your bowels for three to five days. Even if you aren't having pain, you may need treatment for constipation.
- Small stools that are difficult to pass. They can be hard pellets of stool. Patients sometimes tell me that they go every day, but

the colon can still get backed up if you aren't producing enough stool.

- Straining to produce stool. This can be an early warning sign of constipation.
- Abdominal pain or cramping.
- Swollen or distended abdomen as the large intestine becomes impacted, or blocked with stool.
- Nausea or vomiting. If your colon is backed up, the food in your stomach has no place to go.
- In severe cases, patients will say that they have liquid stool or diarrhea. The reason is that only liquid can get around the hard, impacted stool in the left side of the colon.

Sometimes constipation can sneak up on you, and if it's not treated, it can become a serious condition. Recently, I had a patient with metastatic gastric cancer who was experiencing a nagging pain in his lower left side. Dan was seventy-seven years old and his cancer had already spread to his liver, but chemotherapy was doing a good job of keeping the tumors from growing. Because he had some cancer in the right side of his body and in his liver, it was not unexpected that he would have pain on the upper right side of his body. Fortunately, he was able to control this well with a relatively low dose of long-acting oxycodone. But then he was getting an ache in that lower left side. He was able to control it with an additional dose of short-acting oxycodone, but it returned like clockwork whenever the pills wore off. After a couple of days it got worse and became sharp, like a cramp.

Dan called the clinic and I asked him to come in because I was concerned that this new pain might signal an obstruction in his colon. He'd told me that he was moving his bowels every day and urinating every day; aside from the pain, he felt fine. I didn't suspect constipation until I felt his abdomen and it was distended and tender. To determine the cause of constipation, your oncologist will first look at your scans to see whether the cancer is causing it, then look at your medication list because medication is often a cause. Finally, he or she will look at your labs to see whether you are dehydrated, your calcium is high, or your thyroid function is low.

We got some scans for Dan and found air trapped in his bowels by impacted stool. In fact, his entire colon was filled with stool, so much so that it was backing up into the small intestine. At this point a stool softener wasn't going to work, so I had him admitted to the hospital, and we gave him the same liquid that we use to prepare people for a colonoscopy. If you've ever had one of those, you know what GoLYTELY is like. But we didn't have any choice. After about four hours he began to evacuate the entire contents of his colon, and as soon as he did the pain went away. Although this is an extreme example, it shows how serious your medical team is—or should be—about managing your constipation.

Constipation Caused by Medications or Treatment

If you develop constipation, your doctor will be thinking right away that certain medications and conditions of treatment are a likely culprit:

- Opioids for pain
- Anti-nausea medications, particularly the 5HT3 antagonists such as ondansetron (Zofran), palonosetron (Aloxi), and granisetron (Kytril)
- Aluminum-containing antacids such as Maalox
- Calcium channel blockers for high blood pressure, such as diltiazem
- Beta-blockers for high blood pressure, including metoprolol
- Dehydration due to treatment

You'll notice that I've listed no chemotherapy treatments that cause constipation. While it's technically possible for some chemotherapy drugs to cause constipation, it's quite rare.

Most doctors will warn people about constipation, but many people have had no experience with serious constipation before they start cancer treatment. If you've ever been prescribed narcotics for pain after a surgery, particularly orthopedic surgery, then you probably do understand what kind of effect these drugs can have on your bowels. The constipation caused by antiemetics and narcotics can be extremely severe.

Opioids

Nearly everyone who takes an opioid for pain relief will experience constipation. The GI tract has an independent system of active neurons, like those found in the brain and spinal cord. These contain opioid receptors, and, when an opioid binds with them, they slow down the contraction and relaxation phases of peristalsis, and that slows down the whole transit system that's moving food and waste through your body. This includes the anal sphincter, which may be less able to relax enough to let stool pass easily. These opioids also affect the way the body absorbs fluid in the intestines, further making stools dehydrated and harder.

This is why your doctor may give you a recommendation for a moderate to strong laxative alongside the opioid and tell you to start taking the two at the same time. Nobody likes to take extra pills, and some patients claim that they have had good luck with using prune juice or other home-remedy laxatives in their past encounters with constipation. But in many years of treating cancer patients I've found that these natural remedies that may have worked in the past won't work well with opioid-induced constipation. With this kind of constipation, adding fiber to your diet can make stool rock-like and still not move it. It's better to treat this side effect seriously from the beginning with a prescription-strength laxative.

Antinausea Medications

The second major cause of constipation that we see is from the antinausea medications that you take when you get chemotherapy, particularly the 5HT3 antagonists, such as ondansetron and granisetron. I had a patient named Jackson, who was twenty-five when he started treatment for metastatic colon cancer. Jackson experienced such severe constipation from his ondansetron that he developed an anal fissure, which is sort of like a paper cut in the anus, and this made every bowel movement extremely painful. He never told me this, because he was embarrassed, and instead stopped taking his ondansetron for the next infusion. He decided that he would rather suffer through the nausea than risk more constipation. When he finally admitted to me that he was not taking the ondansetron, I got him to a rectal surgeon who got him started on medications to heal the cut. We then had a long talk about other ways to control constipation.

You don't have to give up on your antiemetics and suffer through nausea if you follow a few simple rules. First, always start your laxatives the day before chemotherapy. You want to prime the pump. Second, you have to continue your laxative for one day beyond your final dose of an antinausea drug. So if you are taking an antinausea medication for three days, you'll need the laxative for four days. Remember, too, that mild over-the-counter laxatives almost never work against constipation caused by antinausea medication. You'll need a moderate to strong laxative, usually Miralax or senna.

Aluminum-Containing Antacids

Certain over-the-counter medications can also contribute to constipation, particularly those used to treat stomach acid and acid reflux. I know of one patient who reported that his chemotherapy regimen for lung cancer was causing him heartburn. His doctor couldn't figure out why his constipation was so hard to control, until the patient reported that he was swallowing nearly a bottle of Maalox in the days following every infusion. The active ingredient in Maalox is aluminum hydroxide, which neutralizes gastric acids but it also causes constipation. He switched to a different antacid, Milk of Magnesia. The active ingredient there is magnesium hydroxide, which also neutralizes stomach acid but more often causes loose stools. That small change made all the difference.

Blood Pressure Medications

If you take a calcium channel blocker for high blood pressure, make sure that your primary care doctor knows that you are undergoing cancer treatment, because some of these medications have constipation as a side effect. I had a patient with stage 4 colon cancer who was taking a typical chemotherapy regimen (FOLFOX and bevacizumab). But the bevacizumab was causing her blood pressure to go up, and so her primary care doctor treated her high blood pressure with a standard calcium channel blocker. The next week Mary came into her medical visit complaining of severe constipation. We switched the blood pressure medications to one that doesn't cause constipation, and within two days she was fine. Beta-blockers, which are also often prescribed for high blood pressure, can contribute to constipation as well.

Dehydration

The known side effects from both cancer and treatment include weight loss, nausea, and bowel trouble. Each one of these can contribute to dehydration. The less you eat and drink, the more your GI tract will struggle to work well. The function of the colon is to resorb water from the GI tract. One of the ways that we preserve water when we are dehydrated is increased absorption of water through the colon. So dehydration can lead to a terrible cycle of constipation, where patients don't feel like eating and drinking because they get constipated, which in turn leads to more constipation. That's why your doctors and nurse practitioners will constantly be reminding you to drink.

Older patients may be at high risk for developing dehydration because they are more susceptible to the side effects of minor dehydration, and often their kidney function is not as robust. Your medical team will be urging you to continue to drink fluids even if you aren't hungry and to try to take small meals throughout the day to combat dehydration.

Feeling Constipated, Even When You Aren't

It's possible to have that bloated feeling or cramps even though patients are passing soft stools or even loose stools every day. It's tempting to describe that feeling as the feeling of being constipated. I have had patients who swear that they are constipated even though I've ordered a CT scan that demonstrates no feces in the bowel, and they still don't believe me. These patients aren't constipated in the strict sense of the word, but their brain is telling them otherwise because the cancer is making them feel this way. Some of the following cancer-related conditions can contribute to the feeling of constipation. Others, such as hypercalcemia and hypothyroidism, actually cause constipation:

- Peritoneal carcinomatosis, or abdominal tumors
- Colon obstruction
- Pelvic metastases
- Spinal cord tumor
- Hypercalcemia
- Hypothyroidism

Peritoneal Carcinomatosis, or Abdominal Tumors

This is a common form of metastatic spread where a cancer disseminates throughout your abdomen in little nodules that I often compare to sand or sugar granules. The nodules can eventually grow together and form large clumps of tumor that wrap around the bowels. The presence of these multiple small metastases throughout the abdomen can actually slow down peristalsis, leading to constipation. But just the presence of metastases in the abdomen can activate nerve endings that tell the brain that you are constipated even though you may not actually have any stool in your colon. The presence of tumor nodules can displace these nerves and also cause dysfunctional communication between parts of the nervous system that regulate peristalsis. Furthermore, complex hormonal interactions take place in the GI tract, and cancers can disrupt this process as well. A metastasis anywhere in the pelvis can lead to feeling bloated and constipated. These metastases can press on the colon and cause actual constipation by slowing down bowel movements. Finally, certain spinal tumors can affect the bowels.

Tumor Obstructing the Colon

When a tumor in the abdomen or pelvis wraps around the colon, it both activates nerve endings that tell your brain that you are constipated and causes actual constipation by slowing the transit of stool through that part of the colon. A tumor can eventually lead to a complete obstruction where stool cannot pass. The only way to fix this kind of mechanical obstruction is with a mechanical solution. A surgeon has to remove it or do a bypass operation so that the bowel is redirected around the obstruction. Or a gastroenterologist can place a stent, a tube that is a lot like the coronary stents used to prop open arteries, across the obstruction and open the colon.

Another option is to place an ostomy for stool to exit above the obstruction. A surgeon can bring a loop of healthy intestines to the abdominal wall and create an opening (stoma) through the skin. With an ostomy, your body can eliminate waste into a bag that fits over the stoma. If the surgeon uses the colon, the procedure is called a colostomy. If he or she uses the ileum, the last part of the small intestine, it is called an ileostomy. The stool from an ostomy on the left side of the colon will be well formed, while stool from an ileostomy will be loose and watery. An ostomy can be temporary. If you've had a tumor removed and the surgeon wants the new bowel connection to heal without passing stool, you might need an ostomy for several weeks or months. In other cases, the tumor might cause a complete obstruction that surgeons can't fix, and the ostomy will need to be permanent.

This may sound like a difficult choice, but people learn to live a completely normal life with an ostomy. In fact, nobody ever needs to know that you have one. I had a patient with recurrent small intestinal cancer that was wrapping around her rectum, creating obstruction and causing nausea and pain. Mariana was trying to manage her symptoms with antinausea medicines and pain medicines, but she was completely miserable. After she agreed to undergo a colostomy procedure, she found that her life had changed. She came off of all of her nausea and pain medications. She told me at the clinic that she wished she had done it months earlier.

Hypercalcemia

This is a condition in which your body has unusually high levels of calcium. Cancer patients are at risk for hypercalcemia for multiple reasons. They could have bone metastases, or their cancer cells can produce a substance that mimics the parathyroid hormone, the hormone that regulates calcium. When they get dehydrated from hypercalcemia, they get constipated.

Treating Constipation

Your doctor will treat constipation caused by medication by prescribing laxatives. Table 10.1 below lists the laxatives usually given by strength and how they work to keep the bowels moving. Again, treating constipation is more art than science, and your doctor will give you guidance on how and when to use these medications safely.

If your constipation is caused by the cancer itself, the best way to treat it is by treating the cancer through chemotherapy, surgery, or radiation. Your doctor will likely also prescribe medications to improve stool transit in the short term, until the cancer treatment takes effect.

Laxatives

There are five major classes of laxatives that doctors use in cancer treatment.

TABLE 10.1   *Laxatives by strength and mechanisms*

	Mechanism of action
Mild	
Fruits and vegetables	Bulking agent
Fiber (Metamucil, Citrucel, Benefiber, etc.)	Bulking agent (causes gas)
Docusate (Colace)	Emollient (wets and softens stool)
Dulcolax	Stimulant
Moderate	
Milk of Magnesia	Hyperosmotic
Miralax	Hyperosmotic
Senna	Stimulant
Strong	
Lactulose	Hyperosmotic
Magnesium citrate	Hyperosmotic
Naloxone	Anti-mu receptor

1. Fiber
2. Emollients
3. Stimulants
4. Hyperosmotic laxatives
5. Opioid antagonists

Fiber. These work by bulking up the stool to help move it along the intestinal tract. Examples include Metamucil, Citrucel, and Benefiber. These are great for patients who have had gastrointestinal cancer surgery such as a colectomy. After the surgeon removes a segment of bowel, patients can experience either constipation or diarrhea or both because the colon moves the food through either faster or slower than it did before. Oddly, fiber can help with both of these problems. The only drawback is that people sometimes experience gas or bloating in the first two weeks of taking a fiber supplement. Thankfully, this is usually temporary, and if you can get through those first two weeks, you'll find that fiber helps immensely to regulate your bowels after surgery. The other drawback is that fiber supplements aren't effective in combating the constipation caused by opioids.

Emollients. An emollient is a softening agent. An emollient laxative contains anionic surfactants, such as soaps, that bring more fats and water into the stool and make them easier to pass. The most common example is docusate, also known as Colace. If you take an emollient, you'll notice that your stools will become softer and more liquid. This kind of laxative can be helpful for patients who have anal fissures or hemorrhoids that can be irritated by hard stools. Although highly effective for mild constipation, emollients will rarely be prescribed as the sole laxative to treat constipation caused by opiates or antinausea medications. They are frequently used in conjunction with something else. Vicki often tells patients that emollients create "mush without push," which is why they aren't as useful as other laxatives.

These can also be given as enemas, such as a soap suds enema. These are often difficult for cancer patients to self-administer, but nurses may do this for patients in the hospital or other assisted-living environments.

Stimulants. These drugs help move stool rapidly through the intestines by activating the enteric nervous system and stimulating peristalsis. Bisacodyl (Dulcolax) is one example of a stimulant laxative. These are good for patients with functional constipation, meaning the cancer itself has interfered with or slowed the digestive process. You have to be careful, though, because if you have an actual GI obstruction and the food has no place to go, the stimulants will cause pain and cramping.

Hyperosmotic laxatives. These drugs work by holding more water within the intestinal tract and also drawing water into the GI tract, and they are the mainstay of treatment in the cancer clinic. The stools tend to be watery, almost like diarrhea, but patients can easily modify the dose by how loose their stools are. They are extremely effective against both 5HT3 antagonist and opioid-induced constipation. We will almost always tell patients to start an osmotic laxative prior to using antinausea drugs or an opioid. The most gentle and effective of these is polyethylene glycol (Miralax). And, yes, this is the same substance that is used in most colonoscopy preps, but you will be taking a much lower dose.

Remember that, to take it effectively, you have to drink four to six ounces of water, and this can be difficult for people who are nauseated. Sometimes, against moderate to severe constipation, you need to take a dose two to three times daily. So it's also good to have an extra laxative at the ready. A lot of patients use Milk of Magnesia. You can take two tablespoons (30 cc) every six hours, and this will almost always start the bowels moving and relieve constipation. The process of learning how to control constipation is individual, and you will have to experiment. Sometimes you can tip yourself into having diarrhea. That's why we like to tell patients to start with Miralax alone.

If neither of these works, you should call someone at the cancer clinic who can prescribe something stronger. We often use lactulose, which is a synthetic sugar that causes the colon to retain fluid. It's a syrupy, sweet substance that almost always solves constipation. Some patients don't like it because it's so sweet. Magnesium citrate, a saline laxative, works similarly, and a full glass of magnesium citrate usually induces a bowel movement.

The osmotic agents are almost always effective, but they can be difficult to modify with chemotherapy and narcotics, and thus patients often swing into a day or two of diarrhea. Once you get diarrhea from these agents, stop taking them for twelve to twenty-four hours or until the diarrhea goes away. But if you are on narcotics, you will have to start them again after going twenty-four hours without a bowel movement.

Opioid antagonists. For patients on narcotics, a wonderful anticonstipation drug is naloxone. Naloxone competes with narcotics including hydromorphone, morphine, and oxycodone at the opioid receptors and blocks the effects of the narcotics. In higher doses, emergency responders use it intravenously to counteract effects of a narcotic drug overdose. When taken orally at low doses, it is not absorbed into the system. Instead, it blocks the opioid receptors in the intestinal tract alone. This is a great help to cancer patients taking narcotics for pain because it doesn't block the opioid receptors anywhere in the body except in the GI tract. So your pain medication will still treat the cancer pain, but your stomach and intestines will be free to digest food as usual. Naloxone is unpleasant to take orally, and an injection formulation called methylnaltrexone (Relistor) was created to make it easier to use. This medication is typically given every other day, although some patients don't like to use an injection. You should also know that most insurance companies won't cover this medication unless the patient has tried all the other laxatives and they have not been effective.

Diarrhea

The opposite of constipation is diarrhea, and nearly everyone knows what that's like. But when a physician or nurse practitioner in the cancer clinic asks you whether you are having diarrhea, what they are really asking is whether you have had any increase in bowel movements. These don't need to be the kind of liquid stools people often associate with stomach flu or food poisoning. In fact, they can be semisolid or loose or liquid. Patients are sometimes surprised by how quickly they can move from the constipation caused by antinausea medications to the diarrhea caused by chemotherapy, and it can take a couple of cycles for us to figure out the best course of medications to prevent these swings. For example, I had a twenty-nine-year-old patient with colon cancer who was on a regimen called FOLFIRI, which is a combination of 5-fluorouracil and irinotecan. Both drugs can cause moderate to severe diarrhea, but irinotecan can cause a lot of nausea. Doctors tend to be proactive about controlling nausea in younger patients, because it can be more severe than in older patients, whose brains are less sensitive to chemo-induced nausea. The first time we gave the patient FOLFIRI, we made sure that we also gave him a lot of ondansetron to prevent nausea. It worked well but made him terribly constipated; then when he stopped taking the antinausea drug, diarrhea kicked in from the chemotherapy. The next cycle he started taking Miralax the day before chemotherapy began, which prevented the constipation, but his diarrhea was worse. Within a couple of days, he had to come in and get IV fluids because we were so worried about dehydration. In fact, he wrote me an e-mail where he took Robert Frost's poem "Fire and Ice" ("Some say the world will end in fire / Some say in ice . . .") and substituted "constipation" and "diarrhea." The next cycle we finally got it right by halving the dose of the antiemetics and using half the amount of Miralax. Bowel trouble is no fun, but your doctor will continue to work to find a combination of medications to minimize your discomfort. It's the constant dialog with your medical team that will make the difference.

So, when someone asks whether you are having diarrhea, go beyond a yes or a no. Tell your medical team about the frequency and consistency of your bowel movements, and then compare these to your normal baseline. If your stools are very loose or watery for more than a day, call the clinic. Don't worry about embarrassing anyone, least of all an oncologist or nurse practitioner in a cancer clinic. We are harder to shock than new mothers, in that we talk about poop and vomit all day long.

Some patients can develop more chronic diarrhea from a combination of surgery, chemotherapy, and radiation treatments. I had a patient named Luke who was seventy-four when he started treatment for gastric cancer. He lived about thirty-five miles south of Boston and told me that he developed a Google map with every public

TABLE 10.2 *Major causes of diarrhea*

Cause	Examples
Traditional chemotherapy	Irinotecan
	Fluoropyrimidines (5-FU, TAS 102, Capecitabine)
Targeted agents	Lapatinib
	Erlotinib
	Cetuximab
	Panitumumab
Immuno-oncology	Pembrolizumab
	Nivolomab
Infections	*Clostridium difficile* colitis
	Bacterial overgrowth syndromes
	CMV colitis
Bone marrow transplant	Infections posttransplant
	Graft versus host disease
Antibiotic use	
Bile salt acids after GI surgery	Whipple surgery
	Cholecystectomy
Short bowel syndrome after surgery	
Ischemic colitis	
Tumor infiltration of GI tract	
Overdose of laxatives	
Radiation enteritis	
Neuroendocrine tumors that make diarrhea-causing hormones	

bathroom on the way to the clinic. He would brag that he was never more than five minutes away from any bathroom. He had also acquired ten parking tickets that he successfully defended with doctor's notes from me. I tell patients that bowel conditions like these can be difficult to deal with at first, but you will find a new normal.

In table 10.2, I've listed the various causes of diarrhea.

Treating Diarrhea

Your doctor will have to determine the likely underlying cause of your diarrhea and attempt to treat it. In some cases the fix is easy. For example, if you've taken too many laxatives, that's simple to reverse. If you have an underlying infection, then you will likely take a short course of antibiotics to treat it. Sometimes, when the cause is chemotherapy, the fix is less straightforward. Chemotherapy is often necessary to treat cancer, and, in that case, your doctor will simply try to treat the symptoms alone. Diarrhea needs to be kept under control because it can lead to dehydration and a host of other problems. In fact, you may need IV fluids administered at times when diarrhea is worst. There are four primary drugs that doctors use to treat diarrhea:

1. Imodium (loperamide)
2. Lomotil
3. Tincture of opium
4. Octreotide

Loperamide (Imodium). This is the first line of defense against diarrhea. It's an opioid that doesn't get absorbed into the central nervous system. But it binds with opioid receptors in the intestines and causes the GI tract to slow down. It is available over the counter and comes in two-milligram tablets or capsules. You can safely take a starting dose of two tablets, followed by one tablet every six hours for diarrhea. Sometimes for chemotherapy-induced diarrhea, we ask patients to take one tablet every hour until the diarrhea stops. Generally, it's not recommended to take more than eight tablets a day. If you find that you need to take more or if the diarrhea lasts for more than half a day despite taking hourly loperamide, you need to call your doctor.

Diphenoxylate-Atropine (Lomotil). If loperamide doesn't have a positive effect, then the next drug that we often try is called atropine, or a combination of diphenoxylate and atropine. Diphenoxylate is another opioid-like drug. Unlike loperamide, this drug can be absorbed into the central nervous system and can cause euphoria, but it doesn't control pain very well. Like loperamide, it works primarily in the intestinal tract to slow peristalsis. Manufacturers have combined it with atropine, which can cause tachycardia (a fast heart rate) if taken in high doses. But it can often have a positive antidiarrheal effect where other drugs have failed.

Tincture of opium. This is the next–most aggressive drug we can try if others aren't working. Tincture of opium is also called laudanum or deodorized tincture of opium. Tincture of opium is a very strong antidiarrheal, so strong in fact that it is administered in drops. Doctors use this drug only when Imodium or Lomotil are ineffective.

Octreotide. In patients who are experiencing significant diarrhea from their treatment or cancer, we sometimes use octreotide or one of its analogs. Octreotide is a synthetic imitation of a naturally occurring hormone called somatostatin. This hormone is one of the master hormones that regulate many different actions in the body, including the enteric nervous system. The overwhelming side effect of octreotide is to slow down transit time through the GI tract. It has a number of other effects, including decreasing secretion of fluids by the intestines and pancreas, constricting important blood vessels in the GI tract, reducing gastric motility and peristalsis, reducing the effect of some hormones from the pituitary, and inhibiting contraction of the gall bladder. It's a very useful tool to treat patients who have neuroendocrine tumors that secrete hormones such as serotonin. This is often called carcinoid syndrome, and patients who have it can get overwhelming watery diarrhea. Octreotide is a lifesaver for these patients.

Octreotide can be given intravenously when people are in the hospital, and it can be injected for outpatients. Our favorite form of octreotide is a depot injection, which is a large dose of a drug that is administered as an intramuscular injection (euphemistically called "butt shots" by the general public) and is released into the bloodstream over a four-week period. It sounds painful, but oncology nurses are experts at administering intramuscular injections, and people tolerate them very well. They are administered every four weeks for patient convenience. It can be a wonderful adjunct to the above drugs for patients who suffer from chronic treatment- or cancer-related diarrhea. The only drawback with depot injections is that it takes about two weeks for the drug to take full effect. To bridge the gap, you may need subcutaneous shots (a shot under the skin, the way diabetics self-inject insulin), which can be really uncomfortable.

11

Minimizing Pain

PAIN IS ONE OF THE SYMPTOMS that palliative care specialists and oncologists take the most seriously. Not everyone who has cancer gets pain, but if you do have pain, we want your pain to be well controlled, because living with pain is so exhausting. You can't be yourself and do the things you love to do if you are constantly thinking about pain. And yet, this is the one area where patients seem to struggle the most to communicate how they feel. So many times I hear patients say, "Well, it hurts so much that I can't walk, but I don't want to take anything." Or they say, "I can't sleep at night, but if I take something won't I become an addict?"

You should never expect to live with unmanaged pain, and if your pain is interfering with your daily life, keeping you bedridden, or even keeping you from spending time with your family, you need help.

The experience of pain is intensely personal, something that can make you feel vulnerable and even anxious about the future, and I understand that some people feel uncomfortable talking about it. Many times patients will tell an oncologist—even one they really like and trust—that they have no real problems with pain. Then, on the same day, they come to an appointment with me or with someone in palliative care, and the first subject they want to discuss is how they can't sleep because of the pain or how the medication offered so far isn't helping. When I ask why they didn't bring this up with the oncologist, the answers are often similar:

- "I thought there was supposed to be pain."
- "I don't want him to think I'm weak."
- "What if the cancer is getting worse? I don't want her to stop the chemotherapy."

You should never expect to have poorly controlled pain just because you have cancer, and nobody will think you are weak. While new or increasing pain might be a sign that the cancer is advancing, it might be due to something else entirely. Your oncologist wants to help you manage pain, and most oncologists have training in pain management. But sometimes pain is tricky to manage, and it may require more than one medication or strategy. You have to continue to communicate your symptoms so that the doctor can figure out the right approach to treat not just the pain but the cancer itself. If your doctor has prescribed a pain regimen that isn't working, you need to speak up so that he or she can make adjustments or consult with a pain specialist like a palliative care clinician.

Describing the Intensity of Pain

At every visit to the clinic, someone in your medical team should be asking you whether your pain is acceptable and whether pain is interfering with your normal life. You will be asked whether you have any new pain. This is called a pain assessment. If you do have pain, you will be asked to describe its intensity and qualities. Is it dull or sharp? Can you easily identify the location, or is the pain diffuse? Is it a shooting pain that seems to radiate from one point to another? Does it burn or ache? Is it intermittent or constant? Does it increase or decrease at certain times of day? Is it worse when you move or sit or stand in a certain way?

These are not idle questions. If you develop new areas of discomfort, your doctor needs to know about it. Even if you don't think that

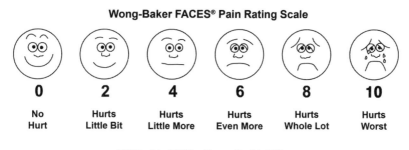

Figure 11.1 Wong-Baker FACES pain rating scale. Wong-Baker FACES Foundation (2015). Wong-Baker FACES® Pain Rating Scale. Retrieved August 19, 2016, with permission from http://www.WongBakerFACES.org.

your pain is related to your cancer, you should still discuss it with your doctor. The sudden emergence of back pain or pain in your bones can alert your medical team to changes in your health. Also, some patients experience pain in areas that have nothing to do with their tumors.

Your doctor will ask you to rate your pain on a scale of 0 to 10 and might present you with a pain scale with numbers and faces on it. Figure 11.1 shows the kind of scale your doctor might use.

This scale is confusing for many people, and some patients are tempted to make their own sad or snarky face whenever presented with it. But doctors understand that pain is subjective, and your sensitivity to pain will be affected by other factors, including your general health, your mood, your level of fatigue. I typically explain it this way: it is unlikely that you will have 0 pain but more likely that we will be able to keep your cancer pain in the 1 to 2 range. The low end of the scale, 1 to 3, represents pain that you notice but that doesn't interfere with your life. With a pain level of 2, most patients can still read the paper or engross themselves in a movie. You can ignore it enough to continue to do almost everything you want. Sometimes your doctor will tell you to treat this pain with over-the-counter analgesics like acetaminophen or ibuprofen. Please don't take these medicines without asking someone on your medical team. There may be reasons your doctor wouldn't want you to treat chronic pain with these types of medications, and there may be better solutions for you.

Moderate pain, between 4 and 6, represents pain that interferes with your daily activities. As part of my pain assessment, I always ask, "Is there anything that you want to do that you can't do because of the pain?" The answer to this question helps me to know how to best treat the pain. Sometimes patients are fine if they are sitting but then have pain when they get up to walk, while other patients have pain that worsens when they are lying in bed, making it difficult to get a good night's sleep. Moderate pain almost always requires treatment with an opioid pain medication such as morphine or oxycodone. Some people are startled by the names of these medications, because they are so often associated with recovery from surgery, but you will likely be starting at a low dose.

If your moderate pain is intermittent, meaning that it comes and goes, you might take an opioid as needed. However, if the pain is constant, your doctor might suggest that you take a short- or long-acting medication on a regular schedule. I am never worried about how much or what type of medication is needed to treat the pain as long as the patient has good pain control and few side effects from the medications.

Severe pain, anything above a 7, is serious and something your doctors will want to treat aggressively. In this situation, you might have a tough time doing anything but think about the pain. Some patients have told me that they have to hold perfectly still or they have to keep pacing to manage the pain. Your team needs to know about this kind of pain immediately. With the right treatments, even severe pain can be made better. Remember, our goal is to get the pain intensity down to that 1 to 2 range. We might not be able to eliminate your pain, but we can reduce it enough to improve your quality of life. Doctors often combine medications and treatments to reduce severe pain.

For example, I met Sarah shortly after she was admitted to Mass General with a diagnosis of breast cancer. Breast cancers tend to metastasize (spread) to the bone, and Sarah was having terrible pain in her left hip from a bone metastasis.

The pain was so bad that she couldn't walk, stand up to shower, or spend time with her family. In fact, she told me that she had to slide herself across the floor to get from one room to another and that her children were really frightened by this. In fact, she cried when she described her children's fears to me. And yet, when I asked her about taking medication for pain, she told me that she thought she should be tough enough to handle the pain, even though the scans revealed that she had a large tumor in the bones of her pelvis.

Before her diagnosis, Sarah had been incredibly active and fit. She played competitively in a women's hockey league two to three times a week. Her children and husband also played hockey. "This is what we do together," she told me. "This is important to me. I want to play hockey again."

I started her on short-acting opioid oxycodone every three hours and ibuprofen every eight hours. This improved her pain in the short term so that she could function more normally. In addition, she started radiation to reduce the pain in her hip. I also started her on a low dose of long-acting oxycodone, which is a pain medication that lasts eight to twelve hours. Most patients with cancer pain need a combination of long- and short-acting pain medications if they have steady pain in addition to acute pain with some activity.

With these medications, Sarah had her pain down to a 2 out of 10. After radiation and some physical therapy, she was able to go back to playing hockey, and she felt like herself again.

Treatments for Pain

Actively engage your medical team about the symptoms of pain and how treatments are working. You can copy table 11.1 and use it to track your symptoms and the effectiveness of any treatments you receive. This will help your medical team assess your dosage and recommend alternatives if your current medication isn't working or has too many side effects.

Nonopioid Pain Relievers

Ibuprofen and naproxen are both nonsteroidal anti-inflammatories, commonly called NSAIDs. These medications can be incredibly helpful in treating any pain caused by inflammation, including bone pain. In truth, most types of pain have some inflammatory component,

TABLE 11.1 *Tracking pain and pain management at home*

Date and time	Pain—location and description	Intensity 0 to 10	Medication taken and dosage	Effect at one hour: Intensity 0 to 10	Nonpharmacologic strategies used (ice, heating pad, relaxation, distraction)

which is why NSAIDs are so often prescribed. You do need to be careful, though. These medications can cause irritation in the stomach and even lead to an ulcer, so they should be used in conjunction with a medication that reduces the stomach's production of acid, such as omeprazole or another proton pump inhibitor. Even with these additional drugs, you can still develop an ulcer. NSAIDs can also affect the kidneys and how they function, so they need to be used very cautiously in patients with kidney problems. Your doctor will want you to monitor for any signs of bleeding while taking an NSAID.

Your clinician will be also looking for other nonopioid treatments for your pain. Acetaminophen can be helpful as an extra medication to treat pain. Other medications such as gabapentin or tricyclic antidepressants can be helpful in the treatment for neuropathic (nerve) pain. These can be prescribed before opioids or in conjunction with opioids.

Short-Acting Opioids

Most patients will require the addition of a short-acting opioid pain medication like morphine or oxycodone to effectively manage cancer-related pain. These medications bind with opioid receptors in areas of the body, including the brain and spinal cord, and reduce your perception of pain. Most short-acting opioids take about an hour to reach peak effect and last somewhere between two and four hours, depending on the intensity of the pain.

If you have intermittent pain or pain associated with a particular activity, you know that the pain might start slowly and peak for a time before it starts to fade. Your doctor may tell you to take a short-acting opioid when the pain starts, so that it increases in effectiveness as the pain increases and then fades roughly when the pain itself will fade. It may be tempting to wait as long as possible before taking the pill, thinking that you should tough it out. But when you do that, you risk doing what we call "overshooting the pain." That means that the opioid takes full effect after the pain has gone away, and that might leave you feeling groggy when you want to be more alert.

One caution using short-acting opioids: it is best to use preparations that do not contain acetaminophen or ibuprofen as a combination product. The reason is that you may need the short-acting opioid every three hours to manage your pain, but it is not safe to take acetaminophen or ibuprofen that frequently. We recommend dosing acetaminophen or ibuprofen separately from the short-acting opioid.

Long-Acting Opioids

If you find yourself taking a short-acting opioid at regular intervals throughout the day, your doctor may suggest that you switch to a long-acting opioid, which is a similar medication but the effects last for many more hours. Table 11.2 lists common long-acting opioids. Many opioids come in a long-acting form. Oxycodone and morphine both have long-acting pills that last eight to twelve hours. These are also known as controlled-release or extended-release oxycodone. Although manufacturers suggest taking a new dose every twelve hours, we have found that it is not uncommon for the pain relief to fall short of the full twelve hours, and you may need to take a new dose after eight. Fentanyl comes in a patch that goes on the skin and typically lasts seventy-two hours. Methadone is another opioid that can be used as a long-acting medication, but it works a bit differently and requires special precautions, so I will describe it in a separate section.

Most often in the outpatient setting we start with medications taken by mouth or patches that are placed on the skin. Many clinicians

TABLE 11.2 *Equivalent IV to oral dosing for opioids*

Opioid	IV	Oral (PO)
Oxycodone	n/a	20 mg
Morphine	10 mg	30 mg
Hydromorphone	1.5 mg	7.5 mg

like to start with oral medications if possible, because it is easier to adjust the dosage as needed. Your doctor may suggest a fentanyl patch if you are having nausea and can't reliably keep down pills or because it is just easier for you to remember to put a patch on every three days rather than taking a pill two or three times per day.

The downside of using a patch is that it can take twelve to twenty-four hours to fully kick in whenever you change the dose. The patch works by seeping into the thin layer of fatty tissue beneath the skin. Patients can struggle to find the right dose if they have lost a great deal of weight during their illness.

Methadone for Pain

Methadone is another long-acting opioid, which you may have heard about as a treatment for heroin addiction. But what you might not know is that it is also an extremely effective, inexpensive, high-potency pain medication sometimes prescribed to treat cancer pain. It may be especially helpful for pain from nerve irritation, the kind that feels like shooting or burning pain.

Methadone is a terrific opioid for severe pain, but it can be very tricky to administer, so you want to make sure that your clinicians have experience prescribing it. Unlike other opioids, methadone takes three to five days to reach peak effect. You and your clinician will need to devise a plan to manage your pain aggressively for those first three days. Your doctor may add steroids to help with the pain for those few days and give you additional short-acting medications. After three days, your doctor can safely increase the methadone.

You never want to overshoot the dose of methadone because it can be unsafe at high levels. I tell patients to be aware of how they feel during those first two days of using methadone. The crazy thing is this: If you feel great on day one or day two, we probably gave you too much. By day three, you could be sleeping all the time if we don't decrease the dose right away.

Remember to take the methadone exactly as prescribed. Never increase your use of methadone without guidance from your clinical team.

Timing Pain Medications

It's sometimes tricky to figure out how to time pain medications, because people are sometimes tempted to hold off as long as they can before taking anything for relief. When I explain the timing of these medications, I sometimes draw a graph on a piece of paper, like the one in figure 11.2. This illustrates the normal ebb and flow of cancer pain through a typical day. There are often normal variations in pain caused by physical movement or other factors, and these are sometimes predictable.

Figure 11.3 shows with shading how the pain medication starts and builds slowly to full effect and then wears off. You can see how the pain medication taken was more than was needed in two out of the four spikes. When you wait to take medication, sometimes the

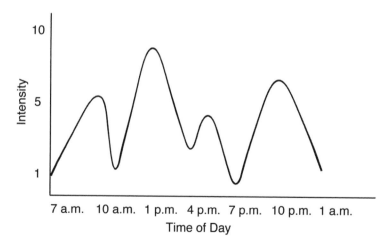

Figure 11.2 Pain without narcotics

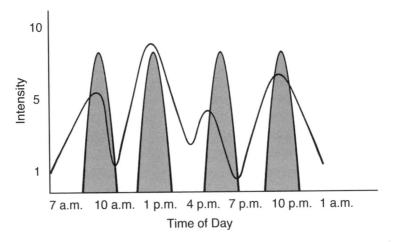

Figure 11.3 Pain with short-acting narcotics; shaded areas indicate pain relief

short-acting medication is reaching peak effect when the pain is less severe. We refer to this as "overshooting the pain" and in that case people experience drowsiness (sedation). It's important to remember that short-acting medications last just three to four hours, so patients can experience erratic pain control.

Long-Acting plus Short-Acting Medication

Patients with chronic cancer pain will always need both a long- and a short-acting opioid. The long-acting opioid treats the baseline pain and provides a constant level of pain relief. It is much more effective because it doesn't cause the peaks and valleys that you get with short-acting pain meds alone. If you just take short-acting pills in succession, you will have peak times when you feel drowsy, and then, as the pill wears off, you will be in a valley with more intense pain until you take the next dose. A long-acting medication will give you moderate pain control all the time, and then you can take an additional short-acting dose when the pain breaks through. This so-called breakthrough pain can happen two or three times per day. If it happens more often than that, we typically use this as a cue to increase the long-acting medication.

A patient of mine, Steve, was really reluctant to start a long-acting opioid. He would say, "I don't need that stuff." He would take the short-acting medication intermittently and as a result alternated between severe pain and sedation. He was too often too miserable to socialize with anyone, and, when he did take pills, he would nod off during conversations. He was sure that starting a long-acting medication would just make that problem worse.

When he finally decided to give it a try, I started him on a low-dose long-acting morphine preparation that he took once in the morning and once in the evening. He felt like a new man. On the scale of 0 to 10, his pain decreased from a 6 to a 3, which was acceptable to him. His sedation was gone, and he had to take a short-acting med only once or twice a day when the pain broke through. I always remind people that in almost every case we can treat pain to bring it down to an acceptable level. Long-acting pain medications can be an important tool in the tool box.

When we start a long-acting opioid, as in figure 11.4, patients experience a much more consistent treatment of their pain. We can still use short-acting opioids for any pain not adequately controlled by the long-acting medication. In general after we start a long-acting opioid, most patients will need the short-acting medication just two to three times per day, as you can see in figure 11.5.

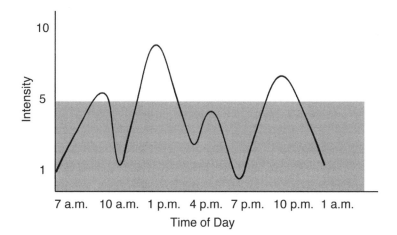

Figure 11.4 Pain with long-acting narcotics; shaded area indicates pain relief

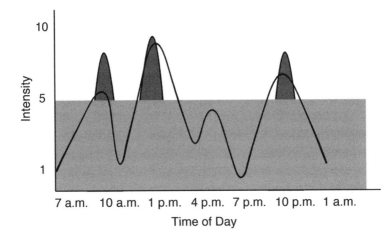

Figure 11.5 Pain with short- and long-acting narcotics; lighter shading indicates pain relief from long-acting medications; darker shading indicates pain relief from short-acting medications

Being Proactive about Pain

A common mistake that patients make is letting the pain get ahead of them. It's tempting to think that you can handle the pain and take care of it later. Patients sometimes tell me that they didn't call the clinic when their pain became disruptive because they didn't want to bother anyone, or they thought they could wait it out until the next medical visit. The trouble is that your pain can escalate over a couple of days, and then it becomes harder to treat.

I suggest that my patients take the short-acting pain medications every three to four hours as needed to keep the pain at an acceptable level so they can do the activities that matter to them. I also advise them to take the long-acting medications as prescribed. Devise a system so you don't forget a dose, because your overall pain control will be worse if you skip doses.

Make sure to track your responses to the pain medication you have been given. You may want to do this in writing or bring someone with you to clinic visits who can talk about your response to pain medication and how it's working. Your medical team wants to know how your pain medications affect you. If the doses make you feel sedated and sleepy when you want to be more active and engaged with your family, your doctor can help you find a better dose for those times of the day. The goal is to have you feeling alert but with good pain control. Sometimes pain can be difficult to manage, and you may need to decide whether you would prefer to have a little more pain but be more alert or have a little less pain and be more sleepy. Sarah, for example, had good pain control for the metastasis in her hip with her oral regimen but experienced sedation. We added a low dose of methylphenidate (a stimulant that is sometimes used to treat ADHD) each morning and at noon, and she was able to have good pain control and still be alert.

Side Effects

Opioids are wonderfully helpful to treat cancer pain, but they can have some side effects that we need to be aware of and manage. These include constipation, nausea, and grogginess. Not everyone experiences all of the side effects. In fact, many of my patients start opioids and don't experience any except for constipation, which is the most persistent side effect.

Constipation is the main side effect you want to be aware of when starting to take an opioid. See chapter 10 for a discussion of the laxatives doctors usually prescribe alongside opioids.

While you may feel groggy or experience some nausea during the first few days of taking an opioid, these feelings should subside within a few days, or a week at most. In those first few days after starting an opioid, I suggest that patients have a medication available to take if they feel any nausea.

Patients also worry about respiratory depression. Opioids are highly unlikely to cause respiratory depression if they are taken as prescribed. Patients who are taking large doses of other sedating medications such as lorazepam and also patients with renal failure, pulmonary issues, or sleep apnea should discuss appropriate dosing with their clinician. Pain can be effectively and safely treated with opioids. You just need to work with your care team to find what works best for you.

Common Concerns

It's normal to be concerned that you may need multiple medications or treatments to reduce your pain. Many patients have asked me whether they will become an addict because they are taking medications sometimes associated with addiction or abuse. Others fear that the medications won't make their life normal, or that they will lose effectiveness over time. Let's take these one by one.

Am I going to become addicted? That's highly unlikely. In the vast majority of cases, cancer patients take opioids effectively just as they are prescribed. These opioids are powerful medications, but the key to avoiding issues related to addiction is to take the medications only as prescribed and to take pain medications for pain only. If you are having anxiety, we should treat it with a medication for anxiety, not a pain medication. Additionally, pain medications help you engage more fully in life. Good pain control means that you can do what you want to do, unlike people with addiction issues, who use opioids to withdraw from life.

Can I drive while taking narcotics? The short answer is no. You should not drive while taking narcotics. The long answer is that people who are on a stable dose of long-acting narcotics for well-established pain might be able to drive without feeling impaired. But this has never been proven. From a legal standpoint, I tell patients that if you do choose to drive and if you cause an accident or injure someone, you may have no legal defense against the accusation that you were impaired.

Will pain medicine make my life normal? The goal of pain medication is to reduce the discomfort that would prevent you from living as fully as you can. Cancer changes your life, and some activities that you used to do may not be possible, but most patients can do a great deal of what they loved before. The key is to reframe your expectations. A patient of mine loves to row crew. He loves to be on the water out there with the other rowers. Then he had a surgery that made getting into a scull hard for several weeks. With aggressive pain control, he could get into a coaching boat with his buddies and be on the water, which he loved. He is still looking ahead to the time when he feels better and in that spirit signed up for a rowing camp that will take place three months after his surgery.

What if they stop working? Another worry that patients have is that pain medications will lose their effectiveness over time. It is true that bodies get more efficient at processing these medications over time—which is called tolerance. Your medical team will know how to compensate to find reasonable pain control. All opioids have different potencies (e.g., 20 mg of oxycodone is equivalent to 7.5 mg of oral hydromorphone). If we find that one opioid isn't working as well as it needs to, you can switch to another. I have had patients who required hundreds of milligrams of opioids per day over the course of several years in order to function. Rest assured your doctor can figure something out. He or she can also refer you to a pain specialist such as a palliative care clinician. We have lots of expertise in managing complex pain syndromes.

Can I just stop taking them? If your pain decreases dramatically, your doctor can reduce the dosage. Do not stop taking opioids abruptly, because you can have rebound pain that is difficult to get under control, and it's possible to have a pain crisis if you stop taking your pain medication suddenly.

Other Strategies for Serious Pain

If you have a sudden, severe onset of pain, your doctor might consider giving pain medication through an IV infusion. Medication delivered in this way typically reaches peak effect in fifteen minutes. You will probably have to be in a hospital setting to receive IV pain medication, but this allows your clinician to quickly figure out how much medication you need and then convert this dosage to an oral regimen you can use at home.

Some patients who need more constant access to IV pain medication can use a PCA, or patient-controlled analgesia pump, that is attached to an IV line. This allows patients to give themselves pain relief as needed. You can just press a button, and the machine will give you a dose of pain medication. Your doctor might suggest this if you are having trouble with oral medications or if your stomach is having trouble absorbing the medication.

These PCA pumps can be portable enough for patients to take them home, if that's necessary. Patients will need to have a longer-term IV, called a PICC line or a portacath, that the medication infuses into, and they will have a small pump for the pain medication to carry with them at all times. It usually fits into a fanny pack.

There are other interventions for pain beyond medication. For some patients, a nerve block can help improve pain control and limit the amount of opioids they need to take. Other patients may benefit from a form of opioid delivery called an intrathecal pump. It delivers pain medication directly to the spinal cord, allowing doctors to prescribe a much lower dose. It does require a trial of the approach to make sure it will work for a particular kind of pain and then a small surgery to implant the pump into the abdomen. It is a great option for certain patients.

Treatments for Localized Pain

When doctors ask patients to describe the pain associated with cancer, they will always ask about location. Is the pain in a defined area, or does it seem to be located inside a bone? Sometimes tumors cause serious pain in a small, well-defined area. If so, your medical team may look to treat that area rather than giving narcotics alone.

Palliative radiation. While radiation is usually given to kill cancer cells and shrink tumors, it has the side benefit of reducing the pain caused by these tumors. And this can be particularly effective if the cancer has metastasized inside a bone. Rather than using radiation to completely remove the tumor, which may not be possible, the treatments can contain it and dramatically reduce the pain it causes. If your doctor thinks you have a metastasis developing in the backbone, he or she will likely suggest radiation as a means of preventing the tumor from reaching the spinal cord. However, if the pain is occurring in multiple sites, radiation may not be the best course of treatment to control it.

Nerve blocks. Another strategy to deal with pain not well controlled by medication is something called a nerve block. An anesthesiologist or pain specialist can inject a substance into or around a nerve to numb it and prevent it from sending pain sensations to the brain. This helps control pain contained in one specific area of the body, and it is often used for people with pancreatic cancer or other cancers in specific organs.

Some people come to the clinic and tell me that they have pain that's exactly like the sciatica they remember experiencing earlier in life. A sharp, shooting pain originating in the lower back and descending down one leg. I have to tell them that this is exactly what they are experiencing. Instead of a disc fragment pressing on the nerve, it's a small tumor. In these cases, a nerve block can be quite effective in controlling the pain.

12

Should I Worry about Shortness of Breath?

THE SENSATION OF BREATHLESSNESS IS one of the side effects of cancer that causes a tremendous amount of worry among patients and their families. Doctors take this side effect seriously as well, and you should talk to your doctor as soon as you begin to feel a change in your breathing. If you find yourself winded going up the stairs or if you can't engage in normal levels of activity without a tightness in your chest or feeling the need to rest to catch your breath, you want to talk to your medical team. Don't worry. There are a lot of strategies your doctor can use to help you breathe easier. Oncologists know that shortness of breath is a side effect that can reduce your appetite and make you less mobile and more isolated. It can also cause anxiety or even a panic attack.

The first thing that people worry about is whether they are able to take in enough oxygen. But in most cases your lungs are fine, and your body is getting enough oxygen. The feeling of breathlessness is actually the feeling that your body is working harder to get air in and out of the lungs. Your diaphragm and chest muscles are working harder to expand and collapse to push the air in and out, and that is what causes the feeling of breathlessness.

Remember that every time you go to the clinic, the medical assistants are taking your vitals, and that includes measuring your respiratory rate and your blood oxygen levels. When patients come into the clinic complaining of shortness of breath, we take those same vitals, and in many cases the oxygen level is fine. Then we know that it's the sensation of working harder to breathe that is the issue.

There are many reasons why cancer can increase your work of breathing:

- If you have not been moving or exercising much, you may be deconditioned and feel out of breath while walking up the stairs.
- In rare cases, chemotherapy can cause a type of inflammation called interstitial pneumonitis, which is swelling in the lining of your lungs, making it difficult to take a full breath.
- You may have pneumonia caused by the cancer blocking one of the bronchi (breathing tubes).
- You could have a blood clot that reduces blood flow to the heart or lungs. Many blood clots are "silent," meaning they don't cause any symptoms, but some can cause inflammation that shuts down the lung.
- You may have low blood counts, meaning there aren't enough red blood cells to carry oxygen to your cells, making you feel that you need to breathe harder even though your lungs are working fine.
- Your abdomen may be filling up with fluid (ascites) or cancer, and it's harder for you to contract and flatten your diaphragm and thus have your lungs fill up with air.
- The space around your lungs may be filling up with fluid (pleural effusion), making it more difficult to move your diaphragm or for your lungs to expand with air.
- Your cancer may have spread to your lungs, and a tumor or spray of small tumors along the lining of your lungs (pleura) may be making it hard for your lungs to expand.
- The cancer may be spreading along the alveoli, the building blocks of the lungs, making it harder for your lungs to expand. This is known as lymphangitic spread.

- Fluid may be building up along the lining of your heart (pericardium), making it more difficult for the heart to move blood through your lungs and making them boggy like a sponge.
- Anxiety or panic can also make you feel short of breath.

Although any one of these causes will interfere with the ease of breathing, none of them usually affect your lungs' ability to take in oxygen, except in severe cases. I had a patient recently with appendiceal cancer that was causing his abdomen to fill up with fluid. Once I told him that his oxygen level was actually fine and that his sensation of working harder to breathe was caused by the fluid pressing against his diaphragm, he seemed relieved. He explained that as a child he had suffered from severe asthma and being short of breath had been a lifelong fear. To cope with the distress, he would sit down and concentrate on breathing slowly and steadily. He had been unknowingly practicing cognitive behavioral therapy (discussed later in this chapter). By slowing down and paying attention to each breath, you can ease the sensation of dyspnea, that is, difficulty breathing, and the anxiety that comes with it.

Diagnosing the Cause

Your doctor may order a chest CT to look for any fluid in the lungs or small tumors. Sometimes you may need an additional test, such as a CT angiogram, also called a pulmonary embolism protocol CT, which uses an IV contrast to check for blood clots in the arteries that feed the lungs. In some cases your doctor may order an echocardiogram, which is an ultrasound that shows how the heart is working. The heart muscle can be damaged by cancer or by chemotherapy, or it may be surrounded by fluid from the cancer, and an echocardiogram is the best way to see whether that has happened.

The results of these tests will determine what may be causing the shortness of breath and give your doctor some idea of how to treat the underlying cause. That might mean draining any accumulating fluid, treating pneumonia, or giving a blood transfusion for low blood counts.

TABLE 12.1 *Causes and treatment of shortness of breath*

Causes	Treatment*
Fluid around the lungs (pleural effusion)	Chest tube and drainage of the fluid
Inflammation in the lung (interstitial pneumonitis)	Steroids
Heart failure	Diuretics
Blood clot (pulmonary embolus)	Blood thinners
Fluid in the abdomen (ascites)	Drainage of fluid
Cancer replacement of lung	Oxygen
Anemia (low hematocrit)	Blood transfusion
Pneumonia	Antibiotics
Deconditioning (being out of shape)	Physical therapy

*After treating any reversible causes, narcotics can be used to ease the feeling of shortness of breath.

The goal of your medical team is to make you comfortable and reduce your anxiety even if the underlying cause of breathing troubles can't be treated. Table 12.1 lists the causes of shortness of breath and the treatments doctors commonly use.

Deconditioning

After you have been in treatment for a while, you may lose weight and avoid some of the activities that you have previously enjoyed. It's a good idea to maintain some level of activity when you are feeling strongest, such as getting out of the house to take a short walk. Without regular walks or movement, your muscles will begin to weaken, and then you are more likely to feel winded when you do move, even though your lungs are working just fine.

One of my patients had multiple surgeries for metastatic renal cell cancer over the course of eighteen months. At the end of this treatment, Paula had no cancer that we could find anywhere in her body, but she complained of being short of breath all the time. I ordered a CT scan of her chest to see whether there was a tumor there or perhaps a blood clot, but the scan showed nothing. Her blood work was fine and so was her oxygenation. Finally, I did what I do with a lot of my patients. I asked her what she thought the problem might be. She said that she thought she might be out of shape. She had never been very athletic, but before her surgeries she had done a lot of gardening and housework and had loved to take long walks.

During treatment she had stopped all of that activity. In fact, she had started using a stair lift to go up and down the stairs. "I just got in a bad habit of sitting around," she said. So I suggested a personal trainer and some more effort with the stairs. A couple of months later she was in the best shape of her life. Of course, you don't have to hire a personal trainer. Even moderate regular exercise can increase your lung capacity.

Pneumonitis

Chemotherapy and radiation can sometimes cause a reaction called interstitial pneumonitis. It sounds scary, but it simply means that white blood cells have infiltrated the lungs and attached to the lining of the alveoli. Doctors treat this with steroids, but these can affect your immune system. This can be tricky if you are taking immunotherapy.

When I was the attending physician on the oncology service in the hospital, one of my patients was using an immunotherapy called pembrolizumab, to treat her melanoma. Pembrolizumab is a PD-1 inhibitor that has been wonderfully effective in treating several types of cancer. But by activating the immune system to attack cancer cells and potential cancer cells, this drug can empower the T-cells (a type of white blood cell, or lymphocyte) in your immune system to attack other kinds of healthy cells. This is what happened to Mariana, who came to the clinic one day panting from the effort of walking into the hospital from the parking lot. When she was checked in, the nurse found that her oxygenation was low. Her oncologist listened to her lungs and heard the telltale crackling sound—like when you first pour milk into Rice Krispies—indicating an inflammation in her lungs, every time she took a breath. The CT scan confirmed this, and she was admitted to the hospital onto my service, and we started steroids to treat the inflammation. We asked a pulmonologist to perform a bronchoscopy (a procedure in which doctors look through a tube down your throat and into your lungs) to get cultures to make sure it wasn't an infection and that I wasn't making the infection worse with steroids, which are immunosuppresive. In her case it wasn't an infection. Three days later, she felt like a new woman. The problem had been that the white blood cells had been attacking the cells lining her lungs, causing her shortness of breath. So we had a balancing act to perform. The steroids can diminish the effectiveness of this cancer treatment. She needed to continue to take the immunotherapy drug to control the cancer along with enough of the steroids to keep the inflammation at bay.

If you do have inflammation in the lungs, your doctor may suggest steroid treatments or inhalers. Many patients can have a component of asthma when they are treated for cancer. You'll know that you are having one of these reactions when you feel yourself wheezing. If your doctor can hear wheezing when listening to your lungs, you might ask for an inhaler similar to those for asthma patients to treat these symptoms.

Pneumonia

Cancer in the lungs can change the way the lungs function, and this can lead to pneumonia. If you have lung cancer or small tumors in the lungs, your doctor may suspect that your shortness of breath may be caused by pneumonia. If you don't have cancer, pneumonia is usually easily treated with a course of antibiotics. When cancer is present, your doctor will check to see whether the tumors may be blocking passageways, which can lead to chronic pneumonia. I remember one patient who came to the clinic with shortness of breath and a fever. A chest X-ray revealed that the airway to the left lower lung (bronchus) was blocked and the pneumonia was behind the blockage. A pulmonary surgeon was able to place a stent (or small tube) in her lung to open up the blockage, and that helped clear up the infection and would hopefully prevent others from occurring.

Blood Clot

Blood clots are extremely common among cancer patients because cancer makes your blood more prone to clotting. These clots typically form along the lining of the veins of the legs and pelvis. They then break off and can go to your lungs. Often, they are silent and we pick them up on routine CT scans. But sometimes they can cause acute chest pain and shortness of breath. We usually treat patients who have blood clots with blood thinners like enoxaparin. Unfortunately, these medications are given by subcutaneous injection (under the skin). Patients have to give themselves these injections once or twice per day, depending upon the drug and the reason for taking it. However, there are new oral drugs that work the same way as the subcutaneous injections. Clinical trials are under way to see if they work just as well as the injections for patients with cancer-related blood clots.

Anemia

When patients are severely anemic, they can feel short of breath, particularly when they move around. The red blood cells carry oxygen to our tissues, and if we don't have enough red blood cells circulating, our muscles don't get enough oxygen. At rest, we have more than enough red blood cells to carry oxygen. But when we exercise or just have a brief episode of extreme exertion like running up a flight of stairs, our muscles, heart, and brain require much more oxygen. If we don't have enough reserve oxygen, we feel short of breath. In every medical visit, someone will take a blood sample and check your red blood cell count. Typically your hematocrit needs to fall under 30 before you will feel short of breath. Normally, our hematocrit runs about 40. So if your red blood count is low, you might benefit from a transfusion or the administration of a subcutaneous injection of erythropoietin, the body's natural hormone that boosts red blood cell production.

Fluid Buildup

As cancer advances, you might have tumors spreading to the lungs and causing a buildup of fluid in the pleural cavity, meaning in the space between the lungs and the thin membrane around the lungs. When fluid accumulates in that space, it prevents your lungs from expanding enough for you to take a full breath.

That's what happened with Sheila, a fifty-eight-year-old woman with breast cancer that had spread to her bones and to the lining of her lungs. She was initially on paclitaxel, a chemotherapy drug that we gave her once a week. Normally, she felt great on chemo, except for numbness and tingling in her hands and feet—a normal side effect for this drug.

Gradually, Sheila noticed that she was short of breath after walking up stairs. When she talked to her doctor, he ordered a chest CT, and it showed more thickening of the pleura, which is the thin membrane around the lungs. This indicated that fluid was accumulating between her chest wall and her lungs, which sounds frightening, but we can drain that fluid. Her doctor ordered a thoracentesis. This is a procedure in which the radiologist numbs an area of skin on your back and puts a needle directly into the space where we see a pocket of fluid to drain it away. In Sheila's case, the radiologist removed a liter of fluid that she then sent to the lab. We do that to check it for cancer cells. After several days the radiologist told Sheila that she did have cancer cells in that fluid, and this shows that the cancer is spreading.

Her doctor switched her to a new chemotherapy drug, called capecitabine, which is a pill rather than an infusion. After several weeks, Sheila noticed that she had more energy and she wasn't getting short of breath as easily. When her doctor did another CT scan, he found that the fluid had disappeared, and she did quite well on this new regimen for many months.

If the fluid is continuously building up, you can undergo repeat thoracenteses to remove the fluid. Your doctor may suggest putting a catheter in place so that you can drain the fluid yourself when you feel short of breath. This may sound a little extreme, but the tubes themselves are thin and flexible, and you can avoid coming to the hospital to have the fluid drained.

Another common procedure is called pleurodesis. For this, your doctor will inject a substance like talc through a chest tube. This substance will cause an inflammatory reaction between the lining of the lung and the chest cavity that essentially seals the lining to the chest wall so that fluid can't accumulate there. Increasingly, catheters are preferred to a pleurodesis, which can be quite painful sometimes and requires a hospitalization.

Supplemental Oxygen

If your blood oxygen levels drop below 90 percent, you might consider getting an oxygen tank to provide supplemental oxygen. Psychologically, it may be difficult to admit that you need extra oxygen, but it might make you feel better and more energetic. And the converse is true as well. If your oxygen saturation is at or above 90 percent, you might not need supplemental oxygen. Some people say that they feel much better when on oxygen, even though it's not raising their oxygen saturation that much. What might also be beneficial in this case is sitting in front of a fan, because it will give you the sensation of taking in more air.

Why Your Doctor Might Suggest Opioid Medications

In some cases your doctor will be able to partially treat the underlying cause of your breathing issues but not all of it. Sometimes the spread of cancer causes this or causes fluids to accumulate after they have been drained. In these cases, your doctor will likely offer an opioid medication to help ease your discomfort. You may need a low dose of an opioid medication to ease the sensation of being short of breath. Opioids work wonderfully to take that feeling away, and you won't necessarily need significant doses. You may feel that you don't want to take an opioid, even a low dose, if you aren't in any physical pain. That's understandable.

My patient Lidia had stage 4 colon cancer that had spread to both lungs. As her lungs gradually began to fill with nodules and fluid, she began to feel short of breath. We put in a catheter to drain the fluid and that helped, but she was still feeling the extra effort to breathe, and it was keeping her up at night. She told me that she had no pain, no problems eating, and no bleeding issues, and she thought that morphine was for junkies. She didn't want to set a bad example for her teenage kids by taking morphine when she didn't feel pain. I totally understood her hesitation but also explained to her that she had made it forty-nine years without getting addicted to anything and that it was extremely unlikely that she would become addicted to morphine. And by taking it, I thought she would sleep better and have more energy for her family during the day. They had a family vacation planned that she was really looking forward to, and I thought she'd have more energy for that, too, if she could sleep better and feel less anxious about her breathing. She finally agreed to give it a try, and the next week couldn't stop telling me how much fun she was having with her boys in the pool.

Another one of my patients was so frustrated by his lack of sleep that he started taking the cough medicine his wife had been prescribed. He told me that he felt dramatically better and was finally able to fall asleep, although it didn't work for very long. Then I told him that the cough syrup contained codeine, which is an opioid. He could continue to take it if he wanted, or I could prescribe a low dose of a long-acting narcotic that would allow him to sleep through the night. He loved it and said he hadn't slept that well in months.

Treating the Anxiety

The other issue your doctor should be asking you about is anxiety. Working harder to breathe causes a lot of anxiety. You are not a wimp because you are feeling anxious about your breathing. It's really important to treat both of these symptoms. We often suggest cognitive behavioral therapy (CBT), which can help you manage the anxiety associated with feeling short of breath.

CBT is a form of psychotherapy in which the patient works with a therapist (typically a psychologist) who looks at the interaction of thoughts and behaviors on feelings. In the case of anxiety from shortness of breath, the therapist will work with you to identify certain thoughts and behaviors that will help mitigate the feeling of anxiety. Cognitive behavioral therapists can help you develop relaxation strategies to reduce anxiety. This might include visualization, such as imagining being on a mountaintop with lots of air moving around you.

These therapists can also help you reframe the sensation of shortness of breath. Many people worry that these sensations are proof that the cancer is getting worse, and they worry that this can't be managed. In truth, there are many treatments that will help.

The CBT clinician will help you work through these fears, and that alone will help you reduce your general anxiety.

There are other techniques you can use to ease the sense of breathlessness. These may include sitting in front of a fan or keeping car windows open while you drive, which helps make your body feel as though it's taking in more air.

Sometimes, anxiety becomes so overwhelming that we need to treat it with medications. Benzodiazepines are wonderful anxiolytics (literally "breaking anxiety") that are quite effective for people with episodic panic attacks. Other medications that can help people feel better with severe anxiety include antidepressants such as citalopram or antipsychotics such as olanzapine.

Can I Die from Being Short of Breath?

Usually, shortness of breath is unrelated to cancer filling up in your lungs and is more often related to an increased *sensation* of shortness of breath because your work of breathing has increased. But it is possible to die of lung failure if the cancer begins to accumulate primarily in your lungs. Sometimes cancers that start in other parts of the body travel to the lungs and spread there. Patients with growing tumors in the lungs often fear that they will not be able to breathe or feel as though they are choking for air. If this is your worry, you will want to talk to your medical team about the steps they can take to avoid this as the lungs become less efficient. Your medical team will continue to remove any accumulating fluid and give you supplemental oxygen. They can also continue to offer medications to control pain and anxiety, and these can make a huge difference.

Sometimes you may need a continuous infusion of pain medication, and we can do that with what we call patient-controlled analgesia (PCA, discussed in chapter 11). It's a portable device that can directly infuse narcotic medication—sometimes morphine or hydromorphone—at a set dose. The device has a second component, which is a button that allows patients to give themselves an extra dose of medication, called a bolus, if needed. You might be familiar with a

PCA if you know someone who has used one while recovering from surgery. You may need to be admitted as an inpatient in the hospital for the medical team to set the appropriate level of pain medication and make you as comfortable as possible before sending you home with a PCA.

13

What If I'm Losing Weight?

SOME WEIGHT LOSS IS NORMAL during the course of chemotherapy. You will likely have days when you feel tired and less like eating. People quickly discover that overeating during treatment can make them feel sick, so they eat smaller meals. Also if you've had surgery, you may come home from the hospital weighing a few pounds less. Most people don't mind this side effect at first. In fact, some of my patients are thrilled, especially if they've struggled with weight gain in the past. They come to appointments excited to tell me that they weigh what they weighed in high school, even though they've lost thirty or forty pounds. They say that they feel healthy and look good. One of the most amazing things that happens when patients lose weight is that their blood pressure and cholesterol levels normalize. If you drop as few as twenty pounds, you may be able to reduce or eliminate your blood pressure and cholesterol medications.

Of course, not everyone feels this way about losing weight. A dramatic change in appearance is an undeniable signal to loved ones that you are dealing with cancer and that your love of food and family meals and cooking has been replaced at least in part by medicines and chemotherapy infusions and side effects. Loss of appetite can be a side effect that causes a lot of tension in a household, and doctors are used to seeing couples fight openly about why the patient isn't eating. It's completely normal to be concerned when a cancer patient doesn't feel like eating much. This situation can trigger worries that the cancer is advancing or that the patient is giving up in some way. But this isn't necessarily the case. Dave and I both spend a great deal of time helping patients and families manage the basic act of taking in calories and all of the emotions that come with it.

Causes of Weight Loss

There are two main reasons for patients to show dramatic weight loss during the course of treatment. The first of these covers a broad group of digestive issues caused by the cancer or the chemotherapy that make eating less appealing or that make digestion less efficient. You may feel less like eating because of nausea, because the taste of food has changed, because your digestive process has slowed, or because of a mass blocking the digestive tract in some way that makes eating uncomfortable. Most of these situations are treatable. The other major reason for weight loss in cancer patients is something called anorexia-cachexia, and researchers don't know exactly what causes it. But it is a progressive weight loss triggered by the cancer itself, and it is not yet treatable except by treating the cancer. There are some promising drugs in clinical trials now, but they have not been approved for general use yet. I will discuss anorexia-cachexia in detail below.

When you come to your doctor asking about how to put weight on or keep it on, you have to know that your medical team can treat some of the issues that contribute to weight loss but not all of them. I'm going to give you some strategies you can use to stimulate your appetite and take in more calories, but some weight loss is hard to treat.

You can use table 13.1 to see how your doctor might work to treat underlying causes of weight loss. Some of these causes have been addressed in other chapters, and some will be addressed in this chapter. A few that may be new are mucositis, pancreatic insufficiency, lactose intolerance, and difficulty swallowing. These are easily treatable

TABLE 13.1   *Underlying causes of weight loss*

Factors that contribute to decreased appetite and weight loss	Possible treatment options
Nausea	Determine the cause of the nausea and aggressively treat. See chapter 9.
Decreased appetite	Dietary changes, appetite stimulants.
Constipation	Goal for bowel movement every day or every other day. Use stimulant laxatives to ensure bowels are moving appropriately. See chapter 10.
Changes in taste and smell	Dietary changes, wait it out.
Early satiety (getting full quickly)	Dietary changes, treat gastroparesis.
Gastroparesis (slow movement of food in stomach)	Use medications that encourage movement of food through the GI tract, for example, metoclopramide, erythromycin. See chapter 10.
Depression	Treat depression with antidepressants that are known to stimulate weight gain, for example, mirtazapine. See chapter 17.
Mucositis	Treat pain associated with the mucositis.
Pancreatic insufficiency	Provide supplemental pancreatic enzymes to help with digestion of food.

in most cases, and, in the case of mucositis, we can treat the pain until the symptoms go away, at which point eating will be more enjoyable again.

Mucositis and Throat Pain

You might already know that chemotherapy can cause mucositis, sores, or thrush in the mouth or throat, and that's why you may be encouraged to chew ice chips or eat a Popsicle during chemotherapy. Keeping the mouth cold during an infusion can reduce the incidence of mouth sores later.

If you have pain when you swallow, this is called odynophagia, and its potential causes include infection, chemotherapy agents, or radiation. Thrush, or oral candidiasis, is a fungal (yeast) infection of the mouth that can be triggered by the steroids you are taking for nausea or the side effects of cancer. It creates white, cottage cheese–like spots on the tongue and mouth. Or if it occurs deeper in the throat, you will notice pain when swallowing. This can be treated with antifungal mouthwashes such as clotrimazole (Mycelex). If this doesn't work, or if it tastes too awful, you can take an oral antifungal called fluconazole that comes in either pill or liquid form. Typically, this kind of infection clears up within forty-eight hours.

Mucositis is harder to treat, but we can reduce the pain while the sores are healing. Your doctor may suggest an oral rinse that will numb the pain and make it easier to eat meals. Oncologists often refer to these rinses as "magic mouthwash," and the recipes for magic mouthwash can vary. Most contain viscous lidocaine, which numbs the nerves of the mouth. It's similar to what your dentist might use before a procedure. Many oral rinses contain lidocaine, Kaopectate, and diphenhydramine (Benadryl) that you swish around in your mouth and then swallow to take away any pain in your mouth and throat. This won't cure the sores—only time will do that—but it will keep the pain at bay. If the pain is severe, you may need additional pain medication.

If you've had cold sores in the past or oral herpes, you may need antiviral medications to treat these sores, which may also emerge after chemotherapy.

Try to avoid foods that will exacerbate the sores. That means no hot and spicy foods, alcohol, or sodas. Also avoid acidic foods, including citrus juices, and coarse foods, including chips, crusty breads, and raw vegetables.

Finally, you want to keep drinking lots of fluids all day long. If you are eating less, you still need to stay hydrated. And you should feel reassured that mucositis and mouth sores will resolve over the course of several days. They come and go with the cycles of chemotherapy. If they are becoming a problem that is affecting the quality of your life, then lowering the dose of chemotherapy is one way to reduce the severity of mucositis.

Difficulty Swallowing

Some patients actually struggle to swallow food or liquids, and doctors call this dysphagia. It can have several causes, including a tumor in the esophagus. If you have trouble swallowing, if food gets stuck, or if you cough a lot after drinking liquids, you should definitely alert your medical team right away. If you are struggling to swallow, you can actually cough your food or drink up into your lungs.

I remember an eighty-five-year-old patient named Olive, who had esophageal cancer. Although her chemotherapy had successfully reduced the size of her tumor, it was still pressing on her esophagus, so she struggled to eat. I helped her choose foods that are easier to get down, and we worked on how to cut up food into pieces that were more manageable. She even found that she could tuck her chin in a particular way to help swallow foods better. Some patients eventually need to undergo a course of radiation therapy to shrink a tumor or to place a tube, or stent, which is a lot like the coronary stents used to prop open arteries, to open up the esophagus to help them pass foods or liquids through. Olive, fortunately, didn't need that. She did fine with chemotherapy and cutting her food into small pieces.

Pancreatic Insufficiency

People with gastrointestinal (GI) cancers can develop something called pancreatic insufficiency. You probably already know that the pancreas regulates blood sugar, but its second major function is to secrete enzymes into the duodenum, the part of the small intestine that helps digest fatty foods. Sometimes cancer or chemotherapy interferes with this second function, and the result is that the body loses the ability to digest fatty foods.

If you have a gastrointestinal cancer and begin to develop loose stools, your doctor may suspect pancreatic insufficiency. Your stools will float in the toilet because of their high fat content. In moderate to severe cases, your stool will look greasy or fatty and smell particularly bad. Don't be afraid to talk about any of this with your doctor because there is a relatively easy fix. You will be given pancreatic enzymes to take with meals. These enzymes aren't absorbed by your stomach but go to work inside your small intestine to help you digest fatty foods.

Everyone has a slightly different diet, and levels of pancreatic insufficiency vary, so you may need to experiment with dosages of these enzymes to relieve the problem.

Lactose Intolerance

As we age, our stomachs lose the ability to make the enzyme lactase, which breaks down the sugars in dairy products. Some chemotherapy interferes with lactase production or exacerbates the normal, progressive lactose intolerance that we all develop over time. And you may have difficulty digesting dairy products. You don't want to be dealing with bloating and diarrhea if you are trying to put on weight or keep it on. So if this happens, you can take lactase pills to alleviate this problem whenever you're eating a dairy product.

Strategies for Keeping Weight On

Many people spend part of their adult lives trying to lose weight by restricting calories, eating salads and other foods that have low caloric density, and avoiding snacks and high-fat foods. When you try to gain or maintain a weight, you have to reverse most of that logic. It sounds fairly simple. The wrinkle is that there will be some days when you want to eat but don't feel up to it because of the chemotherapy, and there might be some foods that you used to love that don't taste right anymore. In fact, even the smell of certain foods might give you an unpleasant reaction. So you have to experiment a little to see what foods you like and what you can safely eat.

Try a wide variety of foods. Some people who used to love sweets find that they really want only savory foods while in treatment. Some people who used to hate spicy foods find them suddenly more appealing. Try new foods to see what works.

Take care of your teeth. Oral hygiene really matters when you are dealing with dysguesia, which is the change in the way foods taste that you get with chemotherapy. Not every patient experiences this. If you do, you need to brush your teeth and tongue every day and floss to keep the problem from getting worse. For whatever reason, dysguesia tends to improve over time. Doctors call this effect the tincture of time. Either you adjust to the new taste of food, or the effect itself wears off over time.

Pay attention to calories. Your goal is to take in 1,500 calories a day, more if you are active. The good news is that there are a lot of calories in butter and soy and full-fat dairy products, as well as nuts and nut butters, so if you can tolerate those, you can have more high-fat foods than anyone you know.

Eat more frequently. Larger meals three times a day are probably not an option when your appetite is not what it normally is. I tell people to eat small meals throughout the day. Your goal is to snack all day in hopes of accumulating calories over time. Don't be discouraged if you can eat just a few bites at a time. In fact, people feel better when they start with an extremely small portion and then take more if they are still hungry. Sometimes facing a huge plate of food is discouraging.

Try energy drink supplements. You can buy these at the store or make your own smoothies with whatever you want—full-fat ice cream, chocolate protein powder. It's up to you. If you can't tolerate milk-based products or don't like the taste of them, you can try some juice-based products or make your own juice smoothies.

Be careful about fiber. Some people who are struggling with constipation may need fiber in their diet to keep things moving, while others who have had GI surgeries or are struggling with loose stools may find that salads and bran products exacerbate the problem. Some patients who loved salads can no longer enjoy them while in treatment. Others are thrilled to say no, finally, to bran muffins.

Avoiding Guilt Trips

I encourage people to practice self-compassion while they are finding new ways to eat. That also means urging family members to be careful about pushing food on cancer patients for their own good. People actually struggle more with eating when they feel pressured. The last thing you want is to have the dinner table become a battleground—even if it's done out of love. I remember a patient, Martha, telling me that her daughter would whip up batches of her famous pudding and then feed it to her by the spoonful, as though she was a toddler. My patient finally put up her hand and said, "Stop. If I am hungry, I'll eat more." Of course, her daughter was hurt and afraid that if she didn't make her mother eat, she wasn't being a good caretaker.

Patients who are losing weight in treatment know that they should eat more, but they are struggling with all kinds of difficulties, including nausea and pain. Sometimes they need to eat very small meals, such as a quarter of a muffin or a few bites of pasta, or they are afraid they will make themselves sick. From the outside, that doesn't seem like enough food. But it's better to respect the patient and to encourage eating without making them feel bad if they can't. It's not realistic to expect cancer patients to eat the way they did before. Sometimes your loved one will want to sit at the table and enjoy the conversation without eating much, and that has to be okay. I tell family members to offer foods they like to eat and leave the rest up to them.

As a patient, you want to be clear with your family that you aren't rejecting the food itself or the love of the people who made it. Educate yourself about nutrition, and experiment with eating different foods you might like in small portions several times a day. Also try to be with those you love when they are eating even if you aren't feeling like eating too much yourself. Meals are such a significant social time for most families.

Doctors are used to seeing couples fight over what the patient is eating and not eating. Dave had a patient, Sammy, who had advanced pancreatic cancer. At every appointment, Sammy's wife would get on him about how little he was eating and how unhealthy he looked, and she would turn pleadingly to Dave to do something. Sammy said that he actually felt fine when he didn't eat, and this would set off an argument each week.

The physical changes of weight loss can be especially hard for spouses. They can feel that this isn't the person they have lived with for decades even though the care team may not see such a dramatic change. This is what happened with Sammy. He later sent Dave a Christmas card of his family. The photo on the front had been taken the previous summer at the Golden Gate Bridge in San Francisco. Dave was stunned by the photo because it showed that Sammy had lost at least fifty pounds since then. Sometimes your care team needs to be reminded of what you see because it is different from what we see.

When weight loss is persistent, everyone needs to remember that the patient isn't eating less because he or she is giving up but rather it is the body's response to the cancer. Preserve meals as a social time to enjoy each other's company.

Appetite Stimulants

Some people are really bothered by their lack of appetite and want to know whether any medications will help. Appetite stimulants don't help patients with metastatic disease (cancer that has spread) to live longer, but some people just want to eat more because they want to feel more normal. That's a good enough reason to give them a try, but be aware of the burdens and benefits of each medication first.

Megestrol acetate contains progesterone and can be helpful to stimulate appetite in some people. However, it can contribute to blood clots. If you are prone to developing blood clots, your doctor will be hesitant to prescribe this drug. Also, the weight that is gained tends to be fat and not muscle. So many physicians will avoid this medication.

Dronabinol is a synthetic cannabinoid. In some states medical marijuana is also available by prescription (described more below). Cannabinoids can increase appetite but often need to be taken several times a day. Many patients experience a high with this medication, which some find pleasant and others find disorienting. I don't like recommending cannabinoids in patients who have a history of psychiatric illness, dementia, or are elderly, as I worry about the risk of confusion and anxiety. We've also been noticing that some of the newer forms of medical marijuana available for patients are much stronger than they were in past years. We caution patients that marijuana isn't a cure-all, and you should discuss your marijuana use with your clinicians.

Olanzapine was created as a treatment for patients with confusion or thought disorders, but there is increasing evidence that it is a powerful antinausea medication and also stimulates appetite and weight gain.

Mirtazapine, an antidepressant and sleep medication, also stimulates hunger in low doses.

Steroids as Appetite Stimulants

Steroids are chemicals that your body already makes in the adrenal glands. Giving additional doses of prednisone or dexamethasone can stimulate both appetite and energy. Even a very low dose of dexamethasone (1 mg per day) can relieve fatigue and stimulate hunger. I had a patient, Delores, who was on a regimen of chemo that required dexamethasone to be given for a day before each infusion and a day after each infusion. This is a common antinausea and antiallergy treatment with some chemotherapy. She said to me that she loved those preinfusion days when she was on steroids. She ate nearly full-sized meals and felt like "the Energizer bunny." Then she switched to a new line of chemo that didn't require steroids. One day in the clinic, she whispered, "What do I have to do to get my hands on some more of that dexamethasone? Thanksgiving is coming and I want to eat!" Whenever patients ask questions like this, I always want to know more about how they truly feel while taking the drug in question. I ask because there are a lot of unpleasant immediate side effects with steroids, including irritability, anxiety or depression, difficulty sleeping, fluid retention, and difficulty controlling blood sugar. Long-term side effects include weight gain, fat deposits in the abdomen and face, muscle weakness, high blood pressure, stomach irritation, and osteoporosis. Even though these side effects tend to occur at higher doses, you can see why doctors are reluctant to prescribe steroids as a long-term solution for patients who just want to eat a bit more.

Still, some patients don't experience any of the difficult side effects at very low doses when they use the medication cautiously. I prescribed Delores one milligram of dexamethasone as needed and told her how sparingly I thought it should be used. She took it the day of Thanksgiving, Christmas Eve, and Christmas Day. At her next appointment, she told me how much she ate and how wonderful it was to feel like herself at the dinner table.

Anorexia-Cachexia

You might continue to lose weight even if you do everything you can to eat enough calories and stimulate your appetite. One major cause of weight loss in cancer patients is something called anorexia-cachexia syndrome. Anorexia means not eating, and cachexia refers to significant loss of weight and muscle mass. People with certain cancers, such as lung and pancreatic cancers, have a higher incidence of this syndrome. It also occurs less commonly with brain tumors or leukemias. Researchers don't yet fully understand what triggers this weight loss, but the suspicion is that some tumors contribute to a production of proteins called cytokines. These cytokines have complicated names such as interleukin-6 and tumor necrosis factor alpha, and they appear to contribute to weight loss in several ways. They seem to increase the body's metabolism, meaning that you need more calories to maintain your weight. They also decrease appetite, making you want to eat less. Finally, they can prevent the body from absorbing nutrients from the foods you do eat. All of these factors make anorexia-cachexia progressive in nature. It's also hard to treat.

Offering nutrition through a feeding tube, for example, might be an excellent way to treat other kinds of nutritional disorders, but, with some kinds of progressive cancer-related weight loss, artificial nutrition doesn't help.

Sometimes patients and families come to the clinic to ask about progressive weight loss when really they are asking a much bigger question about how treatment is going. Weight loss is one of the universal signs that the cancer might be advancing, and it can trigger a lot of worry. When a patient or family member becomes adamant about artificial nutrition or putting on weight, I know that they are often worrying about what this means for them. Patients sometimes start to ask questions about the cancer progressing. This is a good time to start talking with your clinicians about several issues. I like asking patients things like, "What is your body telling you?" "What are your concerns about the future?" "What is good quality of life for you right now?" Many times, people are relieved to give voice to these concerns and to talk about what they truly want for themselves.

Artificial Nutrition

There are two kinds of artificial nutrition. One is enteral, meaning using your stomach (sometimes called a feeding tube), and the other is parenteral, which is giving nutrition through an IV. Doctors prefer to use the gut if they have to give artificial nutrition, but sometimes we don't have a choice and have to use nutrition through an IV.

Some people ask about the possibility of a feeding tube. Enteral nutrition consists of a small tube placed directly into the stomach (called a G-tube, or gastric tube) or the small bowel (called a J-tube, or jejunal tube). This can be done by a surgeon, interventional radiologist, or a gastroenterologist. A nutritionist will then prescribe the best type of nutritional supplement to be administered either as a slow infusion or as a bolus (a larger dose) at regular intervals, which is more like taking in a meal.

In medical school, doctors are taught that the best way to get calories and nutrition into the body is by using the body's system, the stomach and intestines. Doctors tend to suggest enteral nutrition when someone has an obstruction in the duodenum or in the stomach, esophagus, or throat. When you can't swallow food or get it through to your intestines in the natural way, a feeding tube makes perfect sense.

Also, doctors think of enteral nutrition as a temporary solution to the specific problem of taking in calories and nutrition during treatment. If you are undergoing chemo or radiation for the throat or esophagus, for example, you might need enteral nutrition for six to eight weeks to get through the treatment. At the end of treatment, the tube comes out, and you go back to eating regular food.

Parenteral nutrition, or TPN, is given through an IV. It has several drawbacks. Your liver may have problems at first handling the elemental forms of nutrition infused into your bloodstream, so you may have to start slowly. You will probably need to be hooked up to the infusion for a minimum of twelve to sixteen hours a day, which will restrict your movement. The nurses can try to do much of this infusion at night while you are sleeping. If you have a TPN at home, the TPN fluids will have to be delivered to your house and stored there in a specific way. And the tube itself has to be flushed and maintained properly to minimize the risk of infection. But if this is a short-term solution and the benefit is clear, it's worth it.

When Artificial Nutrition Isn't Effective

Putting in a feeding tube becomes tricky when the GI tract is not working well. If your stomach and intestines aren't absorbing nutrition, a feeding tube won't help to improve survival or quality of life. Certain ovarian and gastrointestinal cancers can cause the gut to just stop working. So can peritoneal carcinomatosis, which is the spread of small tumors throughout the abdomen (see chapter 10). In these cases, a feeding tube might actually make patients feel worse because the liquid nutrition sits in the intestines and doesn't get absorbed. We then are faced with the decision to use TPN because intravenous nutrition is the only way. This decision is not as straightforward as it would seem. First, life-threatening infections can occur from TPN. Second, the inconvenience to your daily living of having to administer your TPN can adversely affect your quality of life. Finally, it is the rare patient in which TPN makes a significant positive impact on both survival and quality of life.

Still, there are exceptions, and we are always hopeful that our patients will be the exception. I had a patient with metastatic ovarian cancer that was responding wonderfully to chemotherapy, and yet her GI tract was not working well because of the many surgeries she'd had. She had an appetite for food, but whenever she ate her stomach felt bloated and crampy. She ate smaller meals to feel better and lost 40 pounds. Eventually she was down to 110 pounds, and yet her cancer was responding to the chemotherapy. I suspected that her restrictive diet was the cause of her weight loss rather than the tumors. She was a good candidate for TPN and gained 10 pounds with it, weight that she was able to keep on during the course of her treatment. I would never have recommended the supplemental nutrition if her cancer had been growing out of control. In that case, the risk of harm outweighs any small chance of benefit.

Medical Marijuana

Doctors are often asked about the use of medical marijuana in the setting of cancer treatment. Clinicians have varying opinions on this subject. Some consider the studies of marijuana to treat pain and nausea very compelling, while others worry that the studies that have been done do not show that it is efficacious or even safe in all patients. Some proponents go so far as to say that marijuana can help treat the cancer. Unfortunately, there is no proof behind any of these healing claims with regard to cancer. Marijuana is a product of the cannabis plant, and the psychoactive ingredient is tetrahydrocannabinol, or THC. But THC is one of only hundreds of compounds in marijuana, including many different cannabinoids, the active chemicals in marijuana, and there is a dearth of medical data about what it can or can't do. It has some antinausea, antianxiety, appetite-stimulant, and pain-reducing qualities. One of the problems with marijuana is the variability in purity and the lack of uniform ingredients. There is also very little clinical data to help guide doctors in helping patients make decisions.

The other problem with marijuana is that it's not the best drug for relieving any of the major symptoms in the cancer setting, including nausea, pain, anorexia, and anxiety. Actually, its effect on any of these symptoms can vary greatly from individual to individual. Some people swear by marijuana, and almost every cancer patient has been approached by a well-intentioned friend or family member who pleads with them to try it. Many times, people who used and enjoyed marijuana before they got cancer continue to use it to good effect after their diagnosis. But those people who have never used it before often can't find any value in it once they have a diagnosis. Most doctors are not opposed to the idea of trying it. But Dave often reminds patients that it won't make the cancer better, and that it might not make them feel better if they've never tried it before.

Nutritional Supplements

Lots of patients tell me that they have begun to use various health foods, alternative therapies, and nutritional supplements to augment the cancer treatments they are getting. There is an enormous number of nutritional supplements marketed as cures or preventive measures for every kind of ailment, including cancer. Patients sometimes give me lists of products they are taking and alternate therapies that include coenzyme Q, milk thistle, mushroom extracts, coffee enemas, shark cartilage, high doses of vitamins C, E, and A, as well as teas of every kind. In some cases they just tell me what they are taking, and in other cases they ask me what I think of these supplements. Will they help?

I know that oncologists get these questions, too, and they worry about how to respond. Some oncologists tell me that they just shrug and change the subject. Dave and I like to keep the lines of communication open on this subject, because your medical team needs to know what you are taking and at what doses.

I tell patients that some herbs and supplements do have a pharmacological effect on the body, meaning they can dilute or change the effect of the medications you may be taking to control nausea or pain or other symptoms of cancer—or even the chemotherapy itself. At higher doses, some of them also bring their own side effects, such as a sensitivity in the skin to light, which is a problem for people undergoing radiation, or digestive trouble, or they may even function as anticoagulants in the blood. This is what I tell patients:

- Keep your oncologist and your medical team apprised of what you are taking and at what doses.
- Stay aware of any changes in your body and how you are feeling. You want to report any new side effects or possible interactions between these supplemental therapies and your current medication.
- Keep a critical eye on the science behind the claims for cancer cures. Some websites cite studies that were poorly designed or that have since been disputed.

Also, be careful when mixing and matching large numbers of supplements or alternative therapies. Dave had a patient come to him with a list of twenty different substances he was taking multiple times per day. He was also restricting his diet and undergoing frequent enemas that contained still more substances. Fortunately,

Dave asked two critical questions: "What are you hoping for with these treatments?" and "What do you see as the benefit?" And the patient began to talk about wanting to have some control over the outcome of treatment. He wanted to give himself the best chance at a cure. And then he began to talk more about his anxiety and his inability to talk to his family about what might happen if his upcoming scans didn't show progress. I agree that one of the worst things about having cancer is that sense that you can't control the outcome. Sometimes simply voicing these concerns can provide enormous relief for ongoing anxiety. By contrast, taking large numbers of supplements gives the illusion of control without allowing you to talk about and address your actual concerns.

14

What If I Have a Sudden Fever?

EVERYONE IN A CANCER CLINIC is obsessed with the idea of preventing infection. There are posters everywhere telling you to notify the receptionist if you have a fever or a cough. And you probably notice the way everyone is using the hand sanitizers mounted outside each exam room and along the hallways. There are good reasons for all of this concern. Cancer cells can invade tissues and organs in a way that makes infection more likely to develop. Chemotherapy can also affect your immune system by lowering the rate of neutrophils in your blood, which are the body's first line of defense against infection. These cells help your body kill or neutralize the normally occurring bacteria on your skin, in your mouth and lungs, and in your digestive tract and keep them from entering your bloodstream. As your rate of neutrophils goes down, you are at increased risk of developing infection from bacteria that already exist in your system. In some cases, the port inserted to make chemotherapy infusions easier can become a site of infection. Although a developing infection is a serious condition that requires medical attention, it's also quite common. In most cases, it is also easily treatable.

In this chapter, I'll describe the signs of infection, how your doctor will try to discover the source of the infection, and how most infections are treated. Patients who are receiving a certain type of targeted therapy called immunotherapy are also at higher risk of developing certain types of infections, and you should know about those. I'll also describe the process of bone marrow transplant and how this affects your likelihood of developing infection.

Signs of Infection

The most telling sign of infection is a fever. Always call your doctor if you have a fever of 100.5 degrees or higher or have shaking chills. The higher your fever, the more serious your infection can be. Most adults don't get high fevers, even when they have the flu, and your doctor will suspect that an infection is causing your elevated temperature. While you might have the flu instead, we never assume flu if you have cancer.

If you have chills that cause you to shake, you may be starting to spike a fever. If you have shaking chills, take your temperature right away and then take it again after fifteen minutes.

Other signs of infection include the following:

- Unexpected redness and tenderness on your skin
- Painful urination, which could be a urinary tract infection
- Cough or difficulty breathing
- Sudden onset of confusion, particularly in elderly patients for whom confusion may be the only overt sign of infection

New Symptoms and Infection

These are the most common signs of infection, but if you have any new symptoms, you will want to share them with your doctor. I had a patient once who had a known infection somewhere in his body because he had bacteria in the bloodstream. We did full-body CT scans but found no source. I kept asking him whether he had new symptoms of any kind, and he kept saying no. As he stood up to leave the exam room, he dropped his papers, and I noticed how gingerly he bent down to pick them up. I asked if he was in pain, and he told me that his sciatica was acting up. I asked him why he had never mentioned it, and he told me that he'd had the sciatica for years and that I'd asked for only new symptoms. Fair enough, but I went back to radiology and asked them to take a closer look at one of the tumors that had spread (metastases) to his lower spine and compare it to the previous scans. Did it look different? The radiologist thought that it did. I ordered a biopsy and sent that out for a culture, and it came back positive for bacteria. An infection had developed around the site of the tumor, and that was the cause of his infection. Two days later, a surgeon removed that abscess, and the infection was cured with the help of antibiotics.

Some people may be at higher risk for developing infection during treatment if they've had recurring infections in the past. Vicki had a patient who was just starting to be treated for breast cancer. She felt great during treatment and told Vicki that, aside from the infusions, she could hardly believe she had cancer. On about the ninth day after her third infusion, she told her husband she was suddenly tired and wanted a nap. An hour later, her husband found her asleep and drenched in sweat. She had a temperature of 102 degrees, which is extraordinarily high in an adult. She called the clinic and came in immediately to have her blood drawn. The attending doctor ordered antibiotics for her even before the blood work came back, and when it did come back, it indicated that she had the start of what would have been a runaway infection. Later the patient told Vicki that she'd had a history of urinary tract infections, particularly after sex. So Vicki's sensible advice was to mark a calendar for the seventh, eighth, and ninth days after each infusion and to refrain from sex on those days because the risk of infection is greatest on these days.

Getting Treatment

Infections can be caused by three types of organisms: bacteria, fungi, and viruses. If you have a bacterial infection, which is the most common type, you'll take antibiotics to kill the offending bacteria. Fungal infections usually occur in the setting of a leukemia or lymphoma where the immune system is altered, or when patients have had a prolonged course of steroids. Sometimes fungal infections occur in patients who are debilitated from their cancer. Antifungals do kill the fungi but can require many weeks of treatment to be effective. Viruses, such as herpes or shingles, are treated with antivirals. You may be more prone to reinfection from recurring viruses while in cancer treatment.

You might need several days or weeks of medication to control your infection. However, some patients will need to be on and off these medications indefinitely. In some cases, you will have to come into the hospital for radiation treatments or even surgery to control the infection. The good news is that most infections can be cured or controlled.

It can be tempting to dismiss a slight fever or nagging cough or the sudden onset of fatigue and chills because these seem insignificant compared to many of the other side effects of cancer treatment. It's tempting for anyone to want to take a Tylenol, put on a sweater, or have a nap hoping to feel better in a couple of hours. But cancer is notorious for triggering infections inside the body, and even a small infection can get out of control in a hurry. You can get dangerously sick within a couple of days. If uncontrolled, you can develop sepsis, a condition in which bacteria is in your bloodstream and causes your blood pressure to drop quickly. At that point, you can die of infection. By contrast, if you call the clinic, sit through a blood test, and find out that you really do just have the flu, no one will be upset.

Can I Catch Infection?

People with cancer are always worried about whether they can catch infections from friends, family, or being out in a crowd, and sometimes they ask whether they need to wear a mask. For most patients with cancer, your ability to catch these routine viral infections is about the same as it is for those who don't have cancer, and wearing a mask is generally not helpful. Of course, getting a cold or a flu is not fun even when you are perfectly healthy, so use good judgment in avoiding people who are already sick, and keep hand sanitizer with you while you are out and interacting with other people.

You may wonder too whether you need to take antibiotics before any dental procedures or teeth cleaning. Usually, that's not necessary unless you have a known heart murmur and have always taken this precaution. Theoretically, any hardware inside your body (PICC line or portacath or stent; see chapter 5) can become infected after a dental procedure or cleaning. That's why your doctor might prescribe antibiotics before a dental appointment if you have one of these devices.

Blood Tests and Infection

The main reason your medical team will be closely monitoring your blood counts during every treatment is to monitor your risk of infection. Your level of white blood cells will decrease in the days following each infusion, and you should know that you are more prone to infection about seven to ten days after an infusion, when your white blood count will be lowest.

Whenever your doctor orders a complete blood count (CBC), you should ask him or her to check to see whether your lymphocytes are functioning normally. If they are, then your risk of infection is low because your immune system is likely healthy. If not, your doctor can talk to you about how to avoid the possibility of developing an infection after your infusion. Actually, your chemotherapy might further reduce your chance of getting an infection because it will be attacking the cancer cells that might cause infection.

You should also ask about your level of neutrophils (ANC) after every blood count. This level reveals your underlying risk of infection. Even if your level of neutrophils is high enough for you to receive your infusion, you can still be vulnerable to infection afterward. It's good to know your ANC level, because if you call your doctor or nurse practitioner because you think you might have an infection, it's the first question he or she will ask.

Neutropenia

There will be predictable times during the chemotherapy cycle when you are most at risk for an infection. For most regimens, this occurs seven to ten days after the chemotherapy was administered. Chemotherapy regimens that are given weekly hold a lower risk of infection because the white blood count doesn't get that low.

Most hormonal agents (including antiestrogens such as tamoxifen and antitestosterone agents such as leuprolide [Lupron]) don't carry a significant risk of bone marrow suppression and thus don't carry a significant risk of infection. You can ask your oncologist whether the risk of infection for your specific treatment is low, medium, or high. For patients at high risk of infection, we will often use growth factors to spur on the bone marrow to make more white blood cells.

When your white blood count is low, you may have few overt signs of an infection. Sometimes the only sign that you have an infection is fever. This is known as febrile neutropenia. All the other signs of fever—cough, redness, swelling, or pain—are caused by the white blood cells infiltrating an area in an attempt to fight the infection. When chemotherapy lowers your white blood count, there aren't enough cells to create these other symptoms. That's why getting medical attention immediately is critical. Without treatment, bacteria from the infected area can get into the bloodstream, causing blood infections such as sepsis, septicemia, or bacteremia, which are medical emergencies.

Thankfully, most cases of febrile neutropenia are easily treated. In fact, a few patients come to regard infections as a routine side effect. I was recently serving as the attending doctor in the cancer ward, where I admitted a woman for her eighth episode of febrile neutropenia. She told me that she has a routine where she calls her doctor to tell him that she's febrile again and coming into the hospital. She goes right to the infusion unit and has blood drawn and cultured. The nurses start antibiotics while she waits for a bed to open up. After two days of intravenous antibiotics, her neutrophil level is back above 1,000, and she goes home. She looks great and she told me that she feels great, but she knows she's susceptible to bacterial infections when her blood counts get too low.

Most episodes of febrile neutropenia respond well to antibiotics. If you are at high risk for developing infection, your doctor may prescribe growth factors, which are medications that help boost your neutrophil count.

Treatments That Cause Infection

It's possible for you to develop an infection as the result of a recent surgery. Sometimes the wounds don't heal as they should, and an infection can develop under the tissue as it heals. In that case, you might have to go back into the hospital and have a surgeon reopen the incision to allow the pus to heal directly out of the wound. Radiation treatments can also result in chronic infections. While radiation kills the cancer cells, it can also reduce blood flow to healthy tissue, and, when the tissue doesn't get good blood flow, it can't get access to the white blood cells or antibiotics that kill bacteria, and you can develop chronic wounds and infections.

A common source of infection when patients are on chemotherapy is the catheters and medical hardware that we put in patients to help treat the cancer. For example, the skin overlying the portacath can become infected. Stents that we put into the bowel or the ureters can become infected from the bacteria in your bowel or ureters when the white count gets too low. That's why your doctor will constantly ask you whether you have any indwelling catheters, stents, or any hardware when you have an infection.

Immunotherapy

One of the most exciting advances in cancer care is the development of immunotherapy, in which treatments use the body's own immune system to help kill cancer cells. For decades, researchers studied cancer cells in isolation, wondering why they grow and mutate the way they do. Recently, researchers have focused on the fact that cancer cells don't exist in isolation. They interact with the body's other systems, including the immune system. New research focuses on the ways in which certain cancer cells can essentially fool the immune system into leaving them alone instead of killing them off as defective. This research has yielded some dramatic success stories in particular types of cancer.

One downside of immunotherapies is that they work in a minority of patients. The other downside is that newly empowered immune cells may attack healthy tissues as well, for example, in the tissues in the colon they can cause infections that mimic colitis. If you are undergoing immunotherapy, your doctor will talk to you about the risks of developing these secondary infections and how to manage them.

Infections after Bone Marrow Transplants

Some treatments alter the immune system in profound ways. The most extreme example of this is bone marrow transplantation, which replaces the damaged bone marrow stem cells with healthy cells either from a donor or from your own body. You might need a bone marrow transplant if the treatment requires high doses of chemotherapy that will destroy the bone marrow that creates all of your blood cells. In theory, these high doses of chemotherapy work more effectively against some cancers than do standard doses.

There are two methods for replacing bone marrow: autologous and allogeneic. An autologous transplant is one in which doctors collect your own stem cells circulating in your bloodstream and then replace them after the chemotherapy. Stem cells are the mother cells from which all components of the bone marrow come. So, an autologous procedure is not a transplant in the strict sense of the word, and there won't be any need to search for a donor. Instead, doctors will set up an apheresis machine that looks like one used for a blood transfusion, but it will be collecting the stem cells circulating in your blood to be replaced after chemotherapy.

An allogeneic transplant starts with the high doses of chemotherapy, and then your stem cells are replaced by those of a donor who is genetically similar to you. Both procedures take about two weeks for your infused stem cells to repopulate your bone marrow, and during that time you will be at high risk of developing bacterial and sometimes fungal infections. After your bone marrow is fully functioning, your risk of infection will decline and eventually return to normal.

These new stem cells eventually become your new immune system. The hope is that these new white blood cells will recognize leukemia and lymphoma cells and attack them, while leaving the rest of the body relatively unharmed. We call these transplanted cells the graft cells, and we refer to the patient as the host of these new cells. If these grafted cells attack the normal cells of the host body, we call this graft versus host disease, and it is a possible outcome from transplantation.

If this happens, your oncologist will have to give you immuno-suppressants to weaken your immune system and prevent it from attacking normal cells. But too much immunosuppression may make you prone to infections and also prone to the leukemia and lymphoma coming back. Too little immunosuppression, and you can suffer through terrible graft versus host disease. It really is a balancing act.

When we alter people's immune system with an allogeneic bone marrow transplant, infection is one of the consequences. People can get infections from normal bacteria, atypical bacteria, fungi, and viruses. These infections can be quite severe and even lethal. The oncologists who perform bone marrow transplants are part of their own unique subspecialty. They are more like infectious disease doctors than oncologists in many respects. Ultimately, your graft will take hold, and your body will get used to your new bone marrow. More importantly, your new bone marrow will get used to you. At this point you will get fewer infections and eventually be able to resume a normal life.

Infections from Cancer

Growing tumors are notorious for creating infections. If a tumor grows in such a way that it reduces the blood flow to an organ, an infection will likely follow, and any injury caused by the tumor won't be able to heal properly. Tumors can also block the ducts that drain secretions from organs such as the liver. That's what happened to Amy, who was my patient several years ago. She was in her late fifties and under treatment for pancreatic cancer that was becoming resistant to treatment. She came to the clinic one day with slightly yellowed eyes. Blood tests showed that she had elevated bilirubin, a yellowish substance in the bile produced by the liver, and an ultrasound showed dilated biliary ducts, which help the liver drain waste. The biliary system is like a tree with one long trunk that divides off into two main trunks and then hundreds of small branches. In fact, doctors refer to it as the biliary tree. Unfortunately, the cancer was growing in several places and couldn't be surgically removed. Amy soon developed shaking chills and came back to the clinic, where we found that the blockage had caused an infection. Surgeons were able to put a stent across the duct and open it up, and she felt much better afterward. Still, she continued to develop infections during the next year as the tumors grew, and this is one of the ways that you know the cancer is advancing. You continue to develop infections even though your immune system is working fine. When this happens, your medical team will try to find a way to drain the infection, but this may involve surgery.

Managing Infection as Cancer Progresses

Ron was a seventy-eight-year-old man with lung cancer when I met him as the attending physician on the cancer ward. He had been in treatment for a couple of years when scans revealed that his chemotherapy wasn't holding his cancer steady any longer. Ron had decided to take a break from treatment for a while before deciding whether to enroll in a clinical trial, and, like many patients who take a break, he had immensely enjoyed time away from the infusion unit and the blood tests and the side effects of chemo. He was also looking forward to his youngest daughter's wedding the following month, which is why he had avoided calling the clinic when he developed a persistent cough. The cough kept him up for two nights, but he told his oncologist that he didn't feel short of breath, no more than normal, although he admitted that he wasn't moving around all that much. He was reluctant to come into the clinic for tests because he was afraid that he would be hospitalized and miss the wedding.

His oncologist convinced him to come in for blood tests to rule out an infection, but they revealed an elevated white blood count, and a chest X-ray showed pneumonia. So Ron did have to be admitted for what he hoped would be a short stay. When I examined him a couple of days later, I couldn't hear any sounds at all in that lower quadrant of his left lung, and I ordered a chest CT, which showed that the left lung had collapsed because a tumor had wrapped around the left lower airway. The tumor was preventing him from coughing up the bacteria that was feeding his pneumonia. When a tumor is the cause of this kind of infection, you can take antibiotics to kill some of the bacteria and contain the infection for a little while, but antibiotics alone will never cure it. The bacteria will soon become resistant to antibiotics, and then the infection will spread. Doctors call this a "closed space infection," or abscess, and it's a fairly common scenario as cancer progresses.

Ron and I had a conundrum. I knew that he wanted to attend a wedding in four weeks. The entire nursing staff of the cancer ward knew the date of the wedding, and so did every member of Ron's medical team. We all wanted him to meet his goal of standing up with his daughter on her big day. Yet to give him the best chance of surviving the infection, we needed to figure out a way to open up his lung and drain out the bacteria. Ron wasn't happy to hear any of this. He understood that at his age it was a risk to undergo a surgical procedure, but it was a bigger risk to hope the antibiotics would keep him alive.

Our interventional pulmonologists were able to get a stent into his bronchus to open it up, and then our radiation oncologists recommended radiation to the area to kill the cancer cells that were wrapping around the bronchus. Ron felt a little defeated at first from all of these interventions. He didn't want to have to recover from anesthesia or endure weeks of radiation appointments. No one does. But he did all of it with his goals and values in mind. He knew his priorities and what he was willing to go through to be able to take part in this huge family celebration. When cancer progresses, it's important for patients to be clear about what they want and what they value, because they can better choose the procedures that will be most effective for them.

Can I Die from Infection?

You can die from a runaway infection if it's not treated, and that's why doctors will urge you to be in contact with the clinic constantly about new symptoms and any fevers or shaking chills.

Some patients ask how people ultimately die from cancer, and infection is a common cause of death. Once cancer cells have stopped responding to treatment and are growing through various organs, they are even more likely to cause infections, and those infections become difficult to control without surgery and radiation. Early in your treatment, when the chemotherapy is controlling the cancer, you may be more willing to undergo these interventions, but at some point—months or years from now—you may not. The point is to stay in active discussions with your medical team and your family about your goals for treatment and how many hospitalizations you want to go through.

15

Bleeding and Clotting Issues

THE PROCESS OF CLOTTING AND BLEEDING in your body is an intense balancing act that goes on throughout your life. You don't notice it unless you have a cut or a scrape, but you know it's there. Within minutes of getting a cut on your hand, the bleeding has stopped and the wound is forming a clot. That's because you have proteins circulating in your system with the sole purpose of patrolling for breaks in the vascular system. Platelets arrive first at the site of the cut to plug it, and then clotting factors—proteins responsible for knitting the clot—layer on top of these platelets. If the clot continued to grow, it would clog the blood vessel entirely, and then the tissues on the other side of it wouldn't get the oxygen and nutrients they need. So the body has a competing system of proteins that dissolve clots and prevent them from becoming too big. In medical terms, this process of dissolving clots is called lysis.

As you can imagine, both cancer and cancer treatment can upset this careful balance in the body between clotting and lysis, which is why your doctors will be concerned about the risks of bleeding or developing clots while you are in treatment. It's unsettling to think about these risks, but it's actually routine to have patients dealing with one or the other in the cancer clinic. Your medical team will have a lot of experience in managing these issues.

The Risk of Blood Clots

By far, the most common problem for patients to have is a clotting issue. Many cancers secrete proteins that make it easier for the blood to form clots. It's quite common for patients to develop blood clots, even if they don't realize what's happening. I recently had a patient come in to have routine scans taken. Joanie is fifty-two and has colon cancer but is doing great on chemotherapy, and we expected the scans to show stable disease, meaning no growth in the cancer. An hour after she left the imaging center, I got a page from the radiologist, who wanted to let me know that she had found a pulmonary embolus, or blood clot, in Joanie's lungs. A blood clot in the lungs is considered a medical emergency, so I quickly called Joanie's cell phone to ask how she was doing. She was caught completely off guard by my call and said that she was out having lunch with a friend. Joanie told me that she didn't have any shortness of breath or any pain in her chest. She had no symptoms at all. I asked her to come to the clinic immediately, because whenever we find a clot, we always worry that another, larger blood clot might develop.

If you develop a blood clot, your doctor will probably start you on a blood thinner. Typically, this involves giving yourself a shot under the skin once or twice a day, just as you would if you were a diabetic who needed to self-inject insulin. There are also oral equivalents of these injections in clinical trials now. Doctors are hopeful that these will work just as well and we can replace the shots with pills.

The Dual Risks of Bleeding and Clotting

If you have a blood clot, doctors may want to administer something called tissue plasminogen activator to dissolve it. This is the same substance doctors use on patients who have had a heart attack caused by a blood clot in a coronary artery. Because these clots will damage the heart muscle, doctors know that dissolving the clot is a priority and can save the patient's life.

In cancer treatment, dissolving clots is more complicated because the cancer can be creating clots in one part of the body while invading blood vessels in another part of the body. So you can be at risk for developing blood clots and internal bleeding at the same time. That makes treatment a balancing act of relative risks.

Your doctors are going to be weighing these risks of bleeding and clotting, and they will do so with the best information they have, but sometimes we don't know everything that the cancer is doing inside the body. Another patient, named Todd, had been successfully treated for melanoma. He was doing great until one night he came home from a red-eye flight and became short of breath in the taxi ride home from the airport. He asked to go to the closest emergency room, where a CT scan showed a large pulmonary embolus similar to Julie's. His doctors also administered tissue plasminogen activator to dissolve the clot. As he began to breathe easier, he also had trouble speaking and began to garble his words. With further scans, doctors discovered that Todd had a small brain metastasis, a tumor caused by the melanoma that had spread to his brain, that he didn't know that he had. The tumor had bled into his brain, causing a stroke.

When Do I Call the Clinic?

A little bit of bleeding is common with growing tumors because they require their own blood supply to keep growing. Tumors are made of cells that function almost like ordinary cells. They require a fresh supply of blood and nutrients, and they create their own system of capillaries to obtain these nutrients. As a tumor grows, it will grow through these capillaries and rupture them, causing some bleeding. You may cough a few drops of blood or see small red streaks in your stool. While seeing red blood is always concerning and you should tell your doctor about it, this is usually not life threatening.

Your medical team is going to be more concerned about larger sources of internal bleeding. So if you are coughing up tablespoons of blood or if you see a cup's worth of red blood in the toilet, you need to go to the emergency room to be evaluated. Most people find this hard to judge. If it is more serious, typically people feel sicker. Patients who are bleeding internally often feel weak or faint. Your heart might race even though you are sitting still.

Blood Thinners and Cancer Treatment

If you were being treated for heart disease or blood clots before your diagnosis or if you have had a stroke, your medical team will be talking to you about medications that will help regulate your blood clotting function during treatment. You may spend more time talking to your doctor about the relative risks of bleeding and clotting than does the average cancer patient. Patients often ask whether they can continue to take blood thinners given that some cancers carry a higher risk of serious bleeding. Gastrointestinal (GI) cancers, pancreatic cancer that involves major blood vessels, some head and neck cancers, and liver tumors carry high risks of bleeding.

Your chances of having a bleeding incident will increase as your cancer advances. But these cancers sometimes promote blood clots as well. And any underlying issue such as heart disease, irregular heart rhythms, or lung disease, carries a higher risk that a developing blood clot can be life threatening. It's not unusual in cancer care to have patients who are at risk for bleeding but are also taking blood thinners to prevent clotting. This situation is a complex balancing act, one that you will discuss with your doctor many times. Oncologists often have to weigh whether a patient has a greater risk of dying from clotting or dying from bleeding—but we can often find an answer and adjust your medications accordingly. If you have minor bleeding issues caused by cancer or treatment, you will probably be able to continue using blood thinners. Be aware that if you are on blood thinners and you do experience a bleeding incident that requires a transfusion, your doctor will likely take you off your blood thinners because the risk of severe bleeding has become greater than the risk of forming a clot.

Common Causes of Bleeding

Your body engages in a tightly regulated balancing act of creating and dissolving clots all the time, and that balance can be interrupted by

TABLE 15.1 *Common causes and treatments of major bleeding*

Cause	Treatment
Low platelets	Administer platelets or administer thrombopoietin
Liver failure causing low clotting factors	Medications such as beta-blockers
Cancer causing bleeding by making substances that mimic anticoagulants	Administer blood products and treat the cancer with chemotherapy
Cancer eroding into major blood vessels or organs (fistulas)	Surgery, radiation, or embolization of the cancer
Cancer causing varices to form in the gastrointestinal tract	Injection of antibleeding agents into the varices; treatment of the cancer with radiation

cancer in multiple ways. Cancer treatment can also cause bleeding issues, but doctors will attempt to treat these issues quickly. Table 15.1 lists the major causes of bleeding.

Low Platelets

Having low platelets is commonplace among cancer patients. Sometimes chemotherapy can prevent your bone marrow from making enough platelets, or perhaps the cancer itself is destroying the platelets. Remember that platelets are like the Marines. They're the first ones to attack a cut and stop any major bleeding by laying down the initial aspects of a clot. If you don't have enough platelets or they are not functioning properly, your body will have a hard time forming a blood clot. If this happens, you may have frequent nosebleeds or even see blood in your stool.

Alice had been diagnosed with stage 4 colon cancer and was beginning aggressive chemotherapy to shrink her tumors. Her cancer would bleed from time to time, but she noticed this as a small amount of blood mixed in with her stool. The bleeding always stopped on its own. In addition, she had large external and internal hemorrhoids that had been bleeding on and off throughout adulthood, so we knew that was the cause of some of her bleeding as well. When she started chemotherapy her platelets would drop dramatically after each infusion, and she would notice cupsful of blood in the toilet when she had a bowel movement. She actually needed a transfusion each time this happened to counteract the blood loss. I was able to alter her chemotherapy to prevent her platelets from dropping so much and referred her to a rectal surgeon to treat the hemorrhoids to keep them from bleeding. After her first cycle of treatment, the chemotherapy had shrunk the tumor in her colon enough to keep it from causing bleeding. At that point, the bleeding stopped completely.

Most times when platelet counts are low, the bleeding caused isn't terribly serious, but if your level of platelets gets below 10,000, doctors start to worry about the risk of bleeding into the brain. Thankfully, dropping this low is very rare. If it happens, we can give platelet transfusions to raise the level, and that usually stops the bleeding. Platelet transfusions are effective for a day or two, and in the meantime your doctor will be working to start a treatment for the underlying cause of the low platelet level. For example, if chemotherapy is preventing your bone marrow from making platelets, you might be put on thrombopoietin, which is the growth factor responsible for stimulating the bone marrow to make platelets. If the cancer itself is causing the body to create an antibody that destroys the platelets, the best form of treatment is chemotherapy to kill the cancer. As the tumor cells die, your platelet count will rebound.

In Alice's case, we were able to treat the underlying cancer and adjust the dose of chemotherapy. Sometimes it takes a combination of treatments and a response to therapy to control bleeding. For Alice, this was the beginning of many problems with bleeding over the course of her treatment. Her bone marrow was always especially sensitive to the effects of chemotherapy, and she struggled with low platelets throughout the course of her cancer.

Blood Thinners (Anticoagulants) and Low Clotting Factors

Bleeding can occur when your blood has trouble clotting. If you know someone who takes blood thinners, you know that they have occasional nosebleeds and bruise more easily. Some cancers create substances that mimic the effect of blood thinners. The main way we treat these problems is by treating the cancer. Jamie was a thirty-seven-year-old police officer when she developed intense nosebleeds. Her initial blood tests suggested that she might have a form of hemophilia where the blood lacks a clotting factor. After more tests, her doctor figured out that she had developed an antibody to one of her clotting factors. Realizing that lymphomas can cause this, she had a set of CT scans, which revealed lymphoma in her abdomen. Luckily, it responded nicely to chemotherapy, and as the lymphoma shrunk away she stopped making the antibody to the clotting factor.

It is more common, though, to see patients who are already on blood thinners due to a history of atrial fibrillation or blood clots. People on anticoagulants have a greater risk of bleeding from the medication. Add to that the various risks of bleeding from cancer, chemotherapy, and surgery, and people with cancer are often struggling with bleeding problems.

When Bleeding Is Serious

As cancer advances, there is a greater chance of developing a serious bleeding issue that requires urgent medical intervention. While low platelets and low clotting factors can cause some bleeding, there are other causes of bleeding that are more serious. If you develop tenderness in the abdomen, feel suddenly weak, or have difficulty speaking or any of the traditional signs of a stroke, you also need to contact a doctor immediately.

There are three major causes of internal bleeding: tumors in the gastrointestinal tract, a tumor that erodes into a major blood vessel, and a stroke. Each will require urgent medical intervention, but doctors can often stop the bleeding. It's important to understand how each one of these will be treated if it occurs.

Bleeding in the GI tract. Remember that the stomach and intestines are always contracting to push food and waste along, and the muscles and tissues doing all this contracting require a constant flow of blood to keep working. You have a network of blood vessels and capillaries feeding these tissues, and they are at risk when you have a tumor nearby. Any time a tumor invades these tissues, it can cause a lot of internal bleeding. If you vomit or cough up blood, you will know to call your doctor right away. But another sign of this internal bleeding is a dark, tarry substance in your stool. This substance is what's left of the blood after it has gone all the way through the digestive process. You may also see maroon-colored stool, and that would indicate that the bleeding might be in the lower part of the small intestine or the right side of the colon, and therefore the blood was only partially digested. The first concern for your medical team will be finding the source of the bleeding, so your doctor will be asking a lot of questions about the color of your stool and the amount of blood you've seen. If you have seen a cup or more of blood, your doctors will be concerned that there is massive internal bleeding, and you will probably be admitted to the hospital.

Once you've been admitted, you will probably have an endoscopy, a tube inserted into the GI tract, to find the source of bleeding. An upper endoscopy (or esophagogastroscopy) is when the gastroenterologist places the endoscope into your mouth and down your esophagus. A colonoscopy is when he or she places the endoscope into your anus and up into your colon. Both of these procedures are done while you are asleep. The gastroenterologist may actually be able to stop the bleeding right away, but this is usually a temporary solution. You may have to undergo surgery to stop the bleeding. If surgery isn't an option, you may be able to get radiation treatments that can stop the bleeding for several months. At that point, your doctor will hope that you have a good response to chemotherapy. If the tumor shrinks, the risk of bleeding will decrease as well.

Going through all these interventions may sound like a lot to deal with, but any one of these can stop the bleeding and help you get your life back on track. For example, I had a patient with a ten-centimeter tumor on his pancreas that was invading his stomach. When Paul came to the hospital saying that he had been vomiting blood and seeing tarry stool, we knew he was bleeding a lot. Although surgeons had been unable to remove his tumor, it responded extremely well to radiation, and the bleeding stopped after a few radiation treatments. Because Paul had pancreatic endocrine cancer, which is generally slow growing, he was able to go home with the expectation that it could be years before he would need another such hospital stay.

Another source of serious bleeding in the GI tract is varices. These are dilated blood vessels inside the esophagus or stomach, and you tend to see varices when a vein nearby is partially blocked and the blood vessels leading to that vein get backed up and sometimes rupture under the pressure. As you can imagine, this causes a lot of bleeding. You'll sometimes hear doctors talk about varices as a byproduct of high blood pressure in the portal system. This is confusing to patients, and they will say to me that their blood pressure is normal. Indeed, their blood pressure that we take by the arm cuff is normal. But we mean the blood pressure in the portal system, which is the main venous system of the liver. I had a patient with esophageal cancer that was responding extremely well to chemotherapy when she called to say that she was vomiting blood. Her tumor had shrunk by more than half, and so it didn't make any sense that the tumor would be causing this bleeding. Even the gastroenterologist was puzzled when he did an upper endoscopy and found no bleeding at the site of her tumor. When he looked farther down, he found varices in her stomach. With CT scans, we found metastases in the lymph nodes of her abdomen. These metastases had caused a blood clot to form in a major vein near her spleen. When a surgeon removed it, the varices went away and her bleeding stopped.

Erosion of major blood vessels. The second way that people get serious bleeding is when the cancer is growing in an organ and erodes into a major blood vessel. This is called a fistula, and it wreaks havoc by cutting directly into a vein or artery. This can happen anywhere in the body.

Doctors will typically try to treat this problem with radiation or surgery, depending on the location of the bleeding. One of my patients, Miguel, had metastatic colon cancer that was spreading into his pelvis. He called the clinic to say that he was bleeding from his rectum. A scan revealed that the tumor had eroded into the iliac artery in his pelvis. Fortunately, the surgeon was able to divert the colon around the tumor, and that stopped most of the bleeding. But this kind of issue often requires multiple strategies to stop the bleeding completely. His radiation oncologist was able to radiate the area, and within one week the bleeding had completely stopped. During that week, Miguel received several blood transfusions to keep up his blood count. But it worked, and, after the surgery and radiation, he was able to go back to chemotherapy as though nothing had happened.

Unfortunately, sometimes fistulas are harder to contain. If the tumor is resistant to chemotherapy and radiation, it will continue to erode into major blood vessels. In those cases, we sometimes ask the interventional radiologists to put a catheter into the artery feeding the fistula to embolize it: that is, they inject a substance that essentially blocks off that artery in the same way you would dam an overflowing stream. Embolization is usually a last-ditch effort to stop the bleeding.

Stroke. The third cause of serious bleeding is a stroke. Strokes are caused either by a blood clot going to your brain or by bleeding into your brain. Each is treated very differently. The several risk factors for bleeding in the brain include extremely low platelet counts, blood thinners, or the presence of brain metastases. Radiation to brain metastases will often control the bleeding.

Blood Transfusions

If you have had blood loss after a surgery or bleeding event or if your body is struggling to produce enough red blood cells or platelets because your bone marrow function has been suppressed, your doctor may suggest a blood transfusion as a way to quickly replenish your blood cells. These transfusions are actually fairly common in cancer treatment.

Patients who could benefit from a transfusion might elect to take erythropoietin (epo) instead. This is the naturally occurring growth factor that can boost your body's production of red blood cells. A doctor can administer epo to patients who have chronic bleeding to help them keep up with the blood loss so they don't need a transfusion. A few years ago, a couple of studies tied this drug to an increased rate of blood clots, which meant that doctors stopped using it for a while. Further studies have disputed these findings, and the use of epo now appears to be safe. There are still a number of doctors who are cautious about using it.

Patients who do need a transfusion often ask whether they are at risk for developing infections from donated blood, but the reality is that the risk is extremely low. In a transfusion, you are receiving blood from volunteer donors, but blood banks carefully screen blood.

So the risk of getting HIV from a blood transfusion is 1 in 2.1 million. The risk of being exposed to hepatitis B is about 1 in 275,000, and the risk of hepatitis C is 1 in 1.9 million.

What your medical team will be concerned about is the risk of allergic reaction, which sometimes comes in the form of a fever or rash. Before we administer blood, we always check your ABO blood type and administer the same type of blood. But there are other proteins of lesser importance that are present on the surface of red blood cells. An allergic reaction happens when your body is incompatible with one or more of these lesser proteins and your immune system attacks the red blood cells. In rare instances, this reaction can cause lung injury or other complications. That's why your doctors and nurses will be monitoring your reaction to the transfusion as it happens and for several days afterward, looking for any signs of an adverse reaction. At the first sign of a problem, they will stop the transfusion and treat you for the reaction. Even if this happens, most patients fully recover.

Some people ask whether they can have a friend or family member donate blood to limit the risks of an adverse reaction or infection. You can do this, but there is no evidence that these donations are safer than pooled volunteer donations. In fact, some hospitals discourage these direct donations, however heartfelt, because of the time and effort required to test the blood after it has been collected. All donations, regardless of source, must be screened for infections, including HIV and hepatitis, before they can be used. And donors have to go through the same screening process and questionnaire that they would at a blood bank, and they may have to submit to this process more than once. While friends and family may say that they are eager to help, most doctors have found that this process introduces delays and stress into a situation that is already emotionally fraught. If friends and family members do want to donate blood as a sign of support, they can do so at a blood bank, knowing that they may be saving someone else's life.

16

Why Am I So Exhausted? When
Will I Have Energy Again?

FATIGUE IS BY FAR THE most common symptom patients experience
while in cancer treatment and something we address with all patients in the palliative care clinic. Cancer fatigue is not like any kind
of exhaustion that you've experienced before. It might not improve
much with rest or a good night's sleep. In fact, some patients refer to
fatigue as an unwanted partner in treatment and complain that this
more than anything makes them feel isolated from family and from
the life they used to lead. Some fatigue after each treatment is expected; you may not feel able to do more than rest and sleep in the
days following an infusion. This is normal and your energy level
should rebound day by day.

Someone on your medical team should ask you about your level
of fatigue at every visit to the clinic. The National Comprehensive
Cancer Network publishes guidelines for oncologists on how to provide the best treatment and for patients on how to get the best care.
The NCCN encourages patients to keep an open dialog with doctors
about their fatigue at every infusion because it can so deeply affect
your quality of life. You might want to keep notes, similar to the notes

that you keep on other side effects, so that you can describe your energy level after each treatment and how quickly it rebounds.

Doctors often use a visual analog scale similar to the one for tracking pain. So you will be asked to rate your fatigue on a scale of 0 to 10. Zero means no fatigue at all and 10 indicates the worst fatigue you can ever imagine. Keeping track of how you feel day by day will help your doctors determine whether you are having the episodic fatigue common after an infusion or whether your fatigue is ongoing, which may be caused by other factors, such as medication, sleeplessness, depression, or the cancer itself.

The key is to ask your doctor about any reversible causes and develop strategies to manage your energy effectively. This might involve taking different pain medications, working to get a better night's sleep, or addressing any anxiety or underlying depression. In this chapter, I will go over the most common causes of cancer-related fatigue and strategies to lessen the effects on your day-to-day life.

Episodic versus Ongoing Fatigue

There are going to be some days during treatment where you expect to be tired. If you know that the first two days after an infusion are the ones when you feel wiped out, the fatigue is more manageable, because you can sort of wait it out.

I'm more concerned about ongoing fatigue in which your energy level seems to lag for weeks. If you have fatigue like this that doesn't improve for several days or affects your quality of life in a consistent way, then your care team needs to know. If you were my patient, the first question I would ask is what you want to be doing that you can't do because of the fatigue. Those answers are really revealing. The person who says, "I can't do anything because I feel that I need to sleep all day" is dealing with a totally different problem than is the patient who says, "I used to get through thirty-six holes of golf, and now I can barely do eighteen." If you can't do everything that you used to do, you may be setting expectations too high for yourself while in treatment. By contrast, if you can't do any of the things that you used to do, then there is likely an underlying medical problem that your doctors should address.

The Energy Bank Account

Energy is like a bank account. This is true for everyone, not just cancer patients. You write a check against your energy account whenever you are active throughout the day. You might be doing something pleasant, such as hosting family for a dinner, going shopping, going to the movies, or spending time on your favorite hobby. It could be something less pleasant, such as a stressful meeting or a confrontation, cleaning the house (in my case), or doing anything that's boring but necessary. We all have those tasks in our lives.

When you are in treatment, the balance in your energy account is going to be lower than usual. So it's important to remember that everything you do expends precious energy. I urge patients to choose activities wisely and to make note of those times in the day when they usually have the most energy. Save those high-energy times to do the things that are most fulfilling. If you have a to-do list full of little chores that can be taken care of by someone else, now is your chance to delegate them all without guilt.

This may be a difficult adjustment at first. I have patients say to me that they would never dream of asking someone else to wash their car or mow the lawn or fold laundry. "I don't want to be a burden," is what they tell me. But if you spend a morning doing one of those things, you might not have energy left to spend time with your grandchildren or have coffee with friends.

Some people tell me that they absolutely love scrubbing the grout in the shower or that they find joy in washing the kitchen floor. I don't completely understand this, but if you get excited about dusting the house from top to bottom or detailing your car, then go for it.

Maximizing Your Energy

Running low on energy can be especially frustrating if you are the kind of person who likes to be up and around and doing things and talking to people. It will take time to learn how, but there are several ways you can maximize your energy:

Engage in daily exercise. This doesn't necessarily mean going to a gym or an exercise class. It can be something as simple as a walk every day. Get up and move around so that your muscles have a little bit of strength and stamina.

Get a good night's sleep. Pay attention to how much you are sleeping and what might be interfering with sleep.

Make plans to do something fun. This is an easy one. Spend time with people who make you feel good, and spend the most time doing things you absolutely love. Anticipating fun activities and people to see will give you extra energy during the day.

Causes of Episodic Fatigue

You already know that fatigue is a primary side effect of cancer treatment. Most patients feel this episodic fatigue in the twenty-four to seventy-two hours after an infusion, but it usually diminishes rapidly after those first few days. If your infusions have been scheduled for every two to three weeks, then you will have a week or two to feel more like your old self, but when the infusions occur weekly it can be kind of a grind. Just when you get your strength back, it's time to go back for another infusion. It can feel like a sort of Catch-22. The cancer causes fatigue because it disrupts your body's normal functioning. And the treatment causes fatigue because it is attacking the cancer cells and also disrupting your body's normal functioning. But when the treatments work well, they will actually relieve the fatigue over time. When the tumors are melting away, your energy level will return.

Causes of Ongoing Fatigue

I always encourage patients to keep track of their energy levels over time. A family member or friend can help you remember and note how long it takes for your energy to rebound after a treatment and help track your sleep patterns and what times during the day you have the most energy. This is all good information for planning your time, but it also helps your medical team to figure out what's going on if your fatigue suddenly gets more difficult to manage.

Here are some of the issues your medical team will be thinking about or asking you about if you have ongoing fatigue that doesn't seem to be related to individual treatments.

Have you been on the same course of treatment for several months? Fatigue can accumulate over the course of chemotherapy. If you have had a string of infusions, your energy level may bounce back more slowly over time. A series of radiation treatments can also cause cumulative fatigue that lasts for a couple of weeks after the radiation ends.

Do you have an underlying medical condition? Sudden fatigue can be related to medical conditions other than treatment. This might include low blood counts, which are discussed in chapter 6. The medical term for this is anemia. Your doctor will be following your blood counts closely and will be able to tell right away if this is a problem. If you do have anemia, you might need a blood transfusion.

Fatigue can be a sign of infection, and your doctor will want to rule that out.

Another common medical cause of fatigue is an underactive thyroid gland, also called hypothyroidism. If you already carry this diagnosis, sometimes medications such as iron or calcium supplements can interfere with the absorption of the thyroid replacement medication and make your hypothyroidism worse. There is an easy blood test to check for hypothyroidism so your doctors should rule that out as a treatable cause of severe fatigue.

Rarely, patients can develop adrenal insufficiency if they have been on steroids for a long time. This is true even if you've been taking steroids intermittently with chemotherapy or with drugs like dexamethasone to prevent nausea. Your doctor can pick this up on some routine blood tests but may need to do additional tests to measure your adrenal function.

How much pain are you experiencing? Patients with uncontrolled pain are often exhausted. Many of my patients tell me that they want to take fewer pain medications or want to stay at a lower dose of a medication and then find their pain to be more disruptive than they had anticipated. Experiencing pain all day or all night drains a great deal of energy. I often urge patients to manage their pain more aggressively if they are struggling with fatigue. I have a patient named Will who was having nagging pain in his shoulder after a procedure to treat the tumors in his liver. The tricky thing about pain is that sometimes you experience pain in an area that is not the cause of the problem. In Will's case, he was having what we call "referred pain" in his shoulder from his liver problems. His pain was severe enough to keep him awake at night, and he was miserable and tired all of the time, even though his cancer was responding well to treatment. Will had been reluctant to take any opioids in the past, but then he told me that he and his wife were planning a trip to Paris without the kids. He asked whether there was some way to help him relieve the pain so he could have more energy during his trip. We used a combination of opioids and steroids to reduce his pain, help him sleep, and boost his energy. He and his wife had an amazing time.

What medications are you taking? All kinds of medications can cause fatigue or sedation. Anticholinergic meds such as diphenhydramine (Benadryl) cause you to feel zonked, and you may already know that if the nurses have given this to you as part of your infusion. Patients taking Benadryl during infusions tend to doze off. Gabapentin (Neurontin), which is used to treat neuropathic pain, can also cause sleepiness. Thankfully, this side effect tends to wear off for most people as the body gets used to the medication. So your doctor may suspect that a newly prescribed medication could be causing your fatigue.

Opioids also cause you to feel sleepy. I know I just explained that not controlling your pain aggressively enough can leave you exhausted, and now I have to explain that taking opioids can also drain your energy, particularly during those first few days of taking the medication or the first few days of taking a higher dose. Yet opioids are a mainstay of cancer pain management, so you want to be communicating with your medical team about how well the pills are addressing the pain and how much they are affecting your level of fatigue. With some trial and error, you can find a dose and regimen of pain medication that relieves the discomfort and yet leaves you energetic enough to do the things you enjoy. If you are experiencing a lot of fatigue when you first start taking an opioid, you should know that this won't last forever. You should feel more energy after two to three days as your body gets used to the medication.

Not all opioids are alike in their effects. Short-acting opioids tend to cause more sedation than long-acting opioids. That makes sense because the medications tend to enter the bloodstream quickly, peak in potency after a couple of hours, and then wear off. That's why we use short-acting opioids for managing sudden pain, even though you are more likely to feel fatigue as the medication peaks. Long-acting opioids, by contrast, deliver a more consistent level of analgesia and therefore cause less sedation. So your doctor may want to switch you from multiple doses of short-acting opioid to a couple of doses of a long-acting medication if you have chronic pain and struggle with the fatigue that comes with the medication.

But even with long-acting opioids, I try to be mindful of a medicine's sedative effect when choosing a dosing schedule. For example, long-acting morphine can be dosed every twelve hours or every eight hours. I find that some patients do better with smaller doses divided more frequently. For a patient who requires 120 milligrams of long-acting morphine in a day, I often dose it at 40 milligrams every eight hours rather than 60 milligrams every twelve. Many patients can get more consistent pain control and less sedation with these smaller, more frequent doses.

For patients on larger doses of opioids, cancer fatigue can be treated with methylphenidate (Ritalin). While there is no convincing data that methylphenidate can help with general cancer fatigue, this stimulant can often relieve sedation caused by higher doses of opioids.

Are you eating and drinking enough? Poor hydration and low food intake can contribute to fatigue. What's tricky with cancer is that people often don't feel like eating. Some loss of appetite is normal, and yet there can be a lot of friction within families around how much the patient is or is not eating. Instead of contributing to that friction, I tell patients to just do their best. Eat multiple small meals throughout the day. And remember that you get to eat what you want. This is the time to indulge in full-fat dairy products if you want and put butter on your vegetables. A bigger concern is drinking enough fluids. You might want to keep track of how much water you drink throughout the day to make sure you are getting enough. If you become dehydrated during a difficult chemo regimen, you may need IV fluids intermittently to keep you hydrated and energized.

How well are you sleeping at night? Lack of sleep can make fatigue worse. Unfortunately, a lot of patients struggle to get a good night's sleep. Uncontrolled pain can keep you awake. Certain medications, such as steroids (dexamethasone) used in many chemotherapy regimens, can cause insomnia. And so can anxious thoughts. Many people living with cancer find nighttime particularly difficult. The house is quiet, and there isn't anything to distract you from worrisome thoughts. All of your concerns can sneak up on you at 3 a.m. if you don't have any place to talk about these anxieties during the day. You may find that getting to sleep and staying asleep are challenging, and this will lead directly to daytime fatigue.

I always talk to my patients about what doctors call sleep hygiene, which is all of the habits that contribute to a good night's sleep. They include setting a regular bedtime and preparing for bed by avoiding the television and other screen time late at night. In fact, sleep experts suggest that you use your bed just for sleeping and sex, which may mean removing the television and finding a comfortable chair for nighttime reading. You will want to make sure that the bedroom is quiet, cool, and dark. An air conditioner or fan along with room-darkening shades can help with this.

I also advise patients to avoid naps when they can. On those days when you are wiped out from an infusion or fighting an infection, you can sleep as much as you need to, but on other days I urge people to limit themselves to one 20-minute nap. Set an alarm if you need to. Napping is a big contributor to poor sleep at night. If your body doesn't get a strong enough impulse that it needs sleep, you'll lie awake.

Many people ask whether they should be using medication such as zolpidem (Ambien), lorazepam, trazodone, or melatonin to help with sleep. I think this is a reasonable way to treat insomnia. Some people use these medications only on days when they get steroids in pretreatment, knowing that these steroids will keep them up. Other patients use a slightly higher dose of their regular pain medication at night (such as an opioid or gabapentin) because it helps with pain while also promoting sleep. I also sometimes prescribe other kinds of medications that can be sedating in low doses. These include mirtazapine (Remeron), which is an antidepressant, and olanzapine (Zyprexa), which in higher doses can treat thought disorders but works at low doses to treat anxiety and sleeplessness.

Are you waking early in the morning unable to go back to sleep? If sleeping is an issue, you might want to think more closely about emotional issues that can be disturbing your sleep. Early-morning wakening is a common sign of depression, and your clinician might suggest an antidepressant to help you regulate your mood. Some people don't like the idea of taking an antidepressant, or they think that they take quite enough medications and don't want any more. But I would encourage you to listen to a doctor who suggests that depression may be part of your clinical picture. We know that treating depression is critical to helping patients do as well as possible with their cancer treatment. Patients who are treated for depression do better than those who show signs of depression but refuse treatment.

How are you managing your anxiety? Uncontrolled anxiety can be exhausting. Patients often come to me saying that their fatigue is worse lately, and when we talk more about what's going on, they reveal that they have new concerns about the future or about how treatment is going. Sometimes this new anxiety makes sleep elusive, sometimes it keeps you from exercising, and it can really interfere with doing the activities that you love to do, things that will give you energy. I can't stress enough how important it is to find a safe place to talk about any worries that you have. This is discussed more fully in chapter 17.

If anxiety is keeping you from sleeping, your doctor can prescribe some medications, such as lorazepam, to help you fall asleep. You can also talk to a social worker or psychologist in the cancer center about using relaxation techniques to use when you feel panicked.

Are you exercising regularly? If you are spending large portions of the day in bed or on the couch, your body can become deconditioned, which means that your muscles aren't as strong. Then when you get up and move around, you feel more tired than usual. It's easy for people in treatment to get out of the habit of getting exercise, and then they are surprised when a couple of errands leaves them wiped out. There are going to be some days after an infusion when you really can't get out and exercise, but on those days when you feel a little stronger, you will want to stay active. Aerobic exercises are the most helpful, such as walking or riding a bike. Unless you have a health condition that precludes heart-pumping exercise (such as heart or lung issues) you should try to get about 150 minutes of aerobic exercise per week. You can discuss your exercise regimen with your medical team, but getting more exercise will improve your energy and your quality of life.

For people who have always exercised, this can be an adjustment. One of my patients had been an endurance athlete and exercise fanatic before her diagnosis with metastatic lung cancer at the age of fifty-two. Julie had always loved to go on long runs and spent hours each week at the gym. So, when the tumors that had spread to her brain interfered with her balance and coordination, she stopped exercising, because she was afraid of falling. No more long hikes or eight-mile runs. At first, she felt lost without her exercise routine, but she soon discovered that she could ride a bike just fine and went out on twenty-mile rides every weekend and shorter rides during the week. Julie worked diligently to find that balance between staying safe and getting the exercise she knew her body needed. She did a terrific job of adapting and exercised vigorously throughout her cancer treatment.

Medications for General Fatigue

While several medications work to treat the underlying causes of fatigue, such as pain or sleeplessness, there aren't a lot of medications that are known to specifically relieve the general fatigue that comes along with cancer and treatment. In some cases, I prescribe stimulants such as methylphenidate (Ritalin) or agents that promote wakefulness such as modafinil. The data is not clear that any of these agents significantly improve fatigue, but when we have exhausted all other strategies, it's worth a try.

Another of my patients is Henrietta—Hank to her friends—who often comes to appointments with her husband, Tim. She's in her midfifties and she has colon cancer. She's a great palliative care patient because she's so enthusiastic about life. She's a social worker who is out there fighting for her clients, and when she comes to appointments she's full of questions about managing her sex life and dealing with the ongoing emotional roller coaster of cancer care and managing the pain so she can work as much as possible. We've been working together for about a year and a half now, and she's recently switched to a new line of chemo. It's going well, except for the fatigue. As we talked about this, she said that she didn't have the energy to exercise, and she wasn't sleeping well because she was now worried about the future. It wasn't so much that she wanted to be the life of the party all day, but more that she wanted to have some time during the day when she felt energetic and good.

Hank and I addressed all possible causes. We made sure her blood counts were okay and that she wasn't dehydrated. We got her to exercise about twenty minutes each day, which left her feeling more energized and not depleted. We were sure she wasn't depressed and she was sleeping well, but mornings were still a bear. She just couldn't get herself going and felt like she was a zombie much of the first half of the day. In these situations, it is completely reasonable to try out a medication to increase energy.

A stimulant often works best if we suspect that the fatigue is caused by opioids, but I sometimes try this even when patients aren't on opioids. Methylphenidate is safe for most patients, so talk to your doctor. If you have a cardiac history, he or she may be more cautious in using it, as it can increase heart rate and blood pressure in some patients. Typically I would start with 5 milligrams at 8 a.m. and at noon. Nothing later than 1:00 or 2:00 in the afternoon because taking a stimulant later in the day may interfere with sleep.

Methylphenidate is nice in that it is short acting and lasts about four hours. You don't have to take it every day. You can have it in your toolbox for those days you want an extra boost to feel more like yourself when you go out to lunch with friends. I always tell patients that this isn't going to give them enough energy to run a marathon, but it can offer enough of an energy boost to get out into the world again.

Hank ended up trying some sleep aids so that she could get rest when she needed to. I also gave her methylphenidate each morning and noontime, and she increased her exercise. At our next appointment, Hank said to me, "I feel like I have my life back."

Steroids such as dexamethasone can also increase energy. In fact, some of my patients love being given a steroid as part of their chemotherapy regimen because it gives them so much energy. Steroids are not a great long-term solution because they cause side effects such as ulcers, thinning bones, muscle weakness, and fluid retention. Still, they can be helpful at a low dose given once in a while. I had a patient, Edna, with metastatic lung cancer. She called her dexamethasone her "happy pills" because she was in a much better mood and had increased appetite and much more energy when she took them. In consultation with her oncologist, I gave her a small supply of very low-dose steroid pills that she used for special occasions such as an anniversary dinner or major holiday.

17

Why Do People Keep Asking
Whether I Am Depressed
or Anxious?

IT'S NORMAL TO FEEL ANXIOUS or down while you are being treated for cancer. After all, you are dealing with treatments and side effects along with all of the normal pressures of work and family life. In addition, there may be uncertainty about how well treatments are working and what's going to happen in the future. Any one of these factors can trigger feelings of sadness and loss. While you might be suffering from a clinical depression or anxiety that requires treatment, you might not. In this chapter I will describe ways to distinguish between the common, normal reactions to your diagnosis and signs and symptoms of depression or anxiety that need treatment. Even if what you are experiencing is a normal adjustment to a new reality, that's not going to stop loved ones from asking you about your mood and insisting that you need help with your feelings if you won't talk about them.

Many times in palliative care appointments, I hear from spouses of patients who are determined that a loved one is depressed or needs a therapist or psychiatrist to better deal with emotional issues. I tell lots of patients and their spouses to get away from the notion that someone must be depressed because they have cancer.

Cancer treatment is extremely challenging, both physically and emotionally. Even the process of diagnosis can trigger intense feelings of loss. It is normal to grieve the fact that life is not the same as it used to be. Feeling sad at times is completely normal, and no pill is going to take that away. What's not normal is the feeling that you are always down and that you can't find a way to enjoy your life. It is really important that we treat depression if it exists.

The Difference between Sadness and Depression

Depression is tricky to identify with cancer because so many of the symptoms that signal an acute depressive episode can be caused by the cancer itself. Think about it. The warning signs of depression include loss of sleep and appetite, weight loss, irritability, lack of energy, difficulty concentrating, feelings of helplessness or hopelessness, having negative thoughts, and a diminished interest in normal activities. This checklist is misleading for cancer patients because many of these symptoms can be caused by a cancer diagnosis, by the side effects of cancer, or by the side effects of treatment. And yet, between 15 and 25 percent of cancer patients do experience clinical depression while in treatment. And doctors know from research and from experience that patients who are struggling with depression don't do as well in treatment, so it is crucial to diagnose and treat depression when it is present.

So how do we distinguish between the sadness and grief that's inherent in a big life change from a clinical depression that can affect your health? I always ask patients to talk about the things in their lives that they enjoy. If you were my patient, I would ask how you are spending your time. What do you enjoy doing, and are you taking the time to do it? Are you physically able to do it? Is there any part of your day or your week that you especially look forward to? In part, palliative care professionals ask about your favorite activities so we can help you brainstorm ways for you to live fully, even if some of your symptoms and side effects make these activities more challenging. But we also ask these questions to see how you are getting along generally. We want to know whether you are able to find activities to enjoy and to look forward to.

"I know she's depressed. She needs to talk to someone," is what Gregory said to me about his wife Marta the very first time I met with them. Marta had been diagnosed with non–small cell lung cancer at the age of fifty. She was going through an aggressive course of treatment, and the prognosis was not great, so she did have times when she felt sad and overwhelmed. But when I asked Marta what she enjoyed about her life, she said that she liked going to work. She had built a small advertising business, and she liked being in the office with her partners, seeing the results of different projects. She was also in a fantasy football league, and she loved to obsess about player trades and stats in a way that drove her husband crazy. She wasn't able to do these things every day, but, on the days she felt good, she was working and studying the sports page.

This didn't sound like depression to me. In fact, becoming obsessive about a hobby such as a fantasy league is what I would call a solid coping strategy, something immersive to do when you don't want to think about anything else. The more I talked to Gregory, the more I realized that Marta's illness was having a big impact on his life. I began to wonder whether he would benefit from a place to talk through his worries about the future. It's easy to underestimate how much strain spouses and family members are working under. Sometimes the person demanding therapy for the patient is the one in need of a little extra support. In palliative care, we know that we need to address the needs of the family so that the patient can do as well as possible.

Marta's story was a sharp contrast to that of another patient, Robert, who also had a spouse demanding that he get therapy for his depression. In Robert's case, he had seemed to be coping well with his cancer diagnosis and treatment, and then his wife told me that his mood had fallen off a cliff. At his next appointment I asked him about his golfing buddies, and he said nothing. He was avoiding them. He didn't like to read any more, and he didn't want to spend time with his grandchildren. These feelings persisted even on those days when he was feeling physically strong. I was much more worried that this was a true depression and not just sadness about the cancer. When thinking about mood, doctors don't worry about the fact that you have down days. Everyone does. We worry instead about whether your mood can rebound. When I suspect a clinical depression, I do urge patients to seek treatment, which can be in the form of talk therapy or medication. In the meantime, the first step in feeling better is making sure that your symptoms and side effects are under control.

Uncontrolled Symptoms Affect Mood

Almost any physical symptom can affect your mood. You might feel that you are being strong in not taking much pain medication but then find that the discomfort is sapping your energy or distracting you from doing the simplest activities, such as watching a movie or taking a walk. The same is true with nausea, bowel trouble, insomnia, difficulty eating, or anxiety. Over time, these side effects of treatment can chip away at your resolve, even if you don't think of them as big problems. This is especially true if you haven't felt comfortable talking about them with your oncologist. A terrific benefit of working with palliative care is that we can take the time to ask lots of questions about how you are getting along day to day and find ways to get these problems under control.

For example, I had a patient struggling with severe diarrhea, which was a side effect of her chemotherapy regimen. She hadn't talked much to her oncologist about how bad the diarrhea really was. She was embarrassed to talk about it in detail, which is understandable. Over time, she became fearful of leaving the house because she was afraid that she wouldn't be able to find a bathroom in time. Her life became smaller and smaller until she was showing signs of depression. Once she was able to describe the problem to me, I devised a plan to lessen the impact of the diarrhea in her life. We couldn't eliminate it, but we got her to the point where she could go shopping again and she could go out with her family and visit her friends. Her mood improved dramatically.

Practical Talk Therapy

Perhaps you've tried talk therapy in the past and benefitted from it, or perhaps you are resistant to the idea of talking to a psychologist or social worker about your emotions. Even if you've never tried therapy before, it can really help you cope with the strong emotions that come with a cancer diagnosis. You already know that having cancer isn't like having other problems. It's a different beast entirely, one that complicates all of the relationships in your life, and yet there are many feelings and frustrations that you share with other cancer patients. It's tempting to think that these issues are too big to talk about or that talking alone won't help. But talk therapy can help, particularly if it comes with practical advice and strategies for coping. Research conducted at Mass General has found that patients who engage with a palliative care professional in the early months after diagnosis experienced a 50 percent lower rate of depression compared to other patients. We didn't prescribe more antidepressants. Instead, we gave patients a place to discuss their worries and find things to hope for, and we helped them plan for the future.

I've found that helping patients focus on the future is vital. You may need help finding something to look forward to, something to do that is immersive and meaningful. You want to stay engaged in life, and that can be harder at various points in the process. I find that many patients with serious cancers are afraid to just live. I don't know why, but perhaps it's because everything seems so uncertain. So I try to ask people, "What do you want to do next?" If the answer is a trip to the Grand Canyon with family, I can say, "Great. Let's get your symptoms under control, do some practical planning to make sure you are feeling your best, and buy some travel insurance in case you feel crummy." Patients often tell me that they need to stay optimistic while dealing with cancer, and by that they seem to mean that they have to stay focused on beating the cancer. Instead, I urge people to feel optimistic about enjoying life right now. It's okay to let go and let the clinical team worry about how the treatment is working. One patient said to me, "So let me get this straight. You are going to tell me when I should be more worried about my cancer, and in the meantime, I can just do my thing?" Yes, I said. "That sounds good to me."

You do want to take some care in finding someone who has experience working with cancer patients. If you have the chance to engage with a palliative care professional, you know that this person has a lot of experience helping patients manage symptoms and side effects of cancer and can give solid advice about dealing with it emotionally. You can also ask someone at the hospital or cancer clinic to recommend other therapists with experience treating people who have cancer and all of the unknowns that come with the diagnosis.

A social worker or psychologist can provide an incredibly helpful space to talk through issues more indirectly related to your diagnosis. For example, if you need to talk about getting your ex-husband to be more supportive of your teenage children, a traditional psychotherapeutic relationship might be best. Again, you want to work with someone who understands the unique needs of cancer patients.

Medications

If talking isn't enough, you might consider medication to relieve depression. Some patients tell me that they don't want to take another medication or that they believe that they shouldn't have to take medication for depression. I always say that you are not being a wimp by addressing one of your symptoms. Does it make sense to be going through cancer treatment when you are not at the top of your game? Depression needs to be treated if it affects your life.

I also remind patients that there are lots of options for antidepressants and that these pills are very well tolerated, which means that they bring few side effects. They also work fairly quickly, within two to four weeks, and can have other benefits for cancer patients. For example, some antidepressants increase appetite or help with sleep. Selective serotonin uptake inhibitors (SSRIs) such as citalopram (Celexa) or sertraline (Zoloft) are effective and have few side effects. If the first medication prescribed by your team isn't effective, you have other options. Keep telling your doctor how you are feeling, because it's important to keep depression in check. Table 17.1 lists the common medications used to treat depression.

Anxiety

Cancer treatment brings a lot of anxiety into your life. Of course it does. Who wouldn't be anxious before getting the results from a

TABLE 17.1 *Common medications used to treat depression*

Class	Common drugs in the class	Side effect profile
SSRI Selective serotonin reuptake inhibitor	Fluoxetine (Prozac) Paroxetine (Paxil)* Sertraline (Zoloft) Citalopram (Celexa) Escitalopram (Lexapro)	Generally very well tolerated. Some people can experience dry mouth, diarrhea, and sexual dysfunction. *Paroxetine interacts with many medications prescribed for cancer patients for nausea, etc., so we try to avoid it.
SNRI Serotonin and norepinephrine reuptake inhibitor	Duloxetine (Cymbalta)* Venlafaxine (Effexor XR)	Well tolerated for patients who are not responding to an SSRI. *Duloxetine has been shown to help with neuropathic pain.
NDRI Norepinephrine and dopamine reuptake inhibitors	Buproprion (Wellbutrin)	Buproprion is a helpful medication for patients who have fatigue as a big part of their depressive symptoms. Well tolerated, few to no sexual side effects.
Atypical	Mirtazapine (Remeron)	Sedating, usually given at bedtime to help with sleep. Can also help with appetite.
Tricyclic antidepressants	Nortriptyline (Pamelor) Amitriptyline Doxepin	Most often used in low doses to help with pain or sleep. Used to treat depression only if SSRI, SNRI, etc., have not worked. In the higher doses used to treat depression, we see dry mouth, constipation.
Neuroleptics	Olanzapine (Zyprexa)* Quetiapine (Seroquel)	Being used more to augment the effect of an SSRI or other antidepressant. *Olanzapine is being used more frequently as an antinausea medication, appetite stimulant, antianxiety medication, and for sleep.
MAO-I Monamine oxidase inhibitors	Tranylcypromine (Parnate) Phenelzine (Nardil)	Rarely prescribed unless someone has a life-threatening depression that doesn't respond to anything else. We don't use these often because of many very serious drug and food interactions.

scan? Who doesn't worry about the possibility that the treatment won't work as well as everyone hopes? It's normal to feel anxious about the future. Sometimes the anxiety is going to make it more difficult to concentrate, more difficult to fall asleep at night, more difficult to enjoy some of the ordinary pleasures in life. Some people feel this very real anxiety and then are able to let it go or set it aside for a little while. Maybe they find an engrossing activity or a mindless distraction. Maybe they engage in meditation or prayer. Maybe they've found a place to talk about worries in a way that lessens their impact.

Other people really struggle with anxiety to the point where it affects their day-to-day lives. You want to tell your doctor if your anxiety is keeping you from sleeping or eating or functioning in your life. If you have struggled with anxiety in the past, you may find cancer treatment makes this anxiety worse. Feeling overwhelmed by anxiety is not a failure on your part. I consider anxiety to be a side effect of cancer, and it should be treated as such. The goal is to prevent anxiety from adversely affecting your life each day. You can try some of the coping strategies in chapter 7, or you can try talk therapy, and if you need help for acute anxiety or panic, there are several medications that can help. You can't take all the worries away, but you can lessen them with help.

The Negative Power of Positive Thinking

Many people feel tempted to cope with anxiety by pretending they don't feel it. I find this particularly true for people who say that positive thinking is the key to success in everything. General optimism in life can be incredibly powerful because it helps you take on tough challenges and try new things. Cancer is a different kind of challenge because there are so many aspects you can't control. You can't control the biology of your tumor, and you can't control how effective the treatment is going to be.

Some patients don't want to ever acknowledge that there are things they can't control about their cancer. They feel that this vulnerability will be too overwhelming. Instead, they tell themselves over and over again that they need to stay positive all the time, every minute. Friends and family members can feed this thinking, too, by telling you that you are strong, that you are a warrior, and that you are going to beat this. There is nothing wrong with saying these things or feeling them, but this kind of relentless optimism can actually create anxiety.

I had a patient recently, Julie, who was having a lot of trouble sleeping. She had trouble falling asleep at night and then would wake up at 2:00 or 3:00 in the morning with her mind racing. I asked her what she was thinking about when she couldn't sleep, but she didn't want to tell me at first. Finally, she admitted that she was worrying about what would happen if her cancer got worse. She worried about her husband and how he would care for her if she were really sick, and how she would be letting him down if she didn't get better. Then she sat up straighter and said, "But I can't think like that. I have to stay positive." She wasn't really talking to me at that point. She was lecturing herself. She also said that if she didn't stay optimistic, she was inviting her cancer to grow.

I hear this a lot, and I know that optimism can be an useful tool to help you cope with a crummy situation. But it's not healthy to police your thoughts all the time or to completely deny the normal fears and negative thoughts that come with a serious diagnosis. Negative thoughts can't be pushed aside forever. If you deny them, they pop up when you least expect them, usually in the middle of the night. In palliative care, we encourage people to talk about their worries, to talk about what might happen if the cancer gets worse, even if they can only do so for a few minutes at a time. We do this because it is another great tool for coping. By acknowledging your worries, you lessen their control over you.

I worked with Julie on this, asking the questions that I ask all of my patients:

- What has your oncologist said about what might happen in the future?
- When you think about the future, what do you think about?
- What do you worry might happen?
- What if one of the things you worry about did happen? What would that be like?

- Can we think of some strategies for how you would cope with this if it did happen?
- How can your family get support if something like this did happen?

Allowing yourself to talk about what might happen and what you worry about doesn't invite your cancer to get worse. It's just another conversation that falls under the heading "What If." While you can have these conversations with a palliative care professional, you can also have them with a close friend or family member or a therapist experienced with cancer treatment.

At first it was difficult for Julie to admit to the things that she worried most about. These conversations take practice. Over time she found that she could describe more of her concerns about the future. She wondered how much longer she could work. She worried that if she stopped working, she wouldn't be able to afford college for her kids. She worried about who would care for her aging mother. She wondered aloud if she could really die from her cancer. These are enormous concerns, and yet she hadn't talked to anyone about them. Her need to stay positive had actually isolated her from her family and prevented her from thinking of any practical solutions. We talked about the possibility of her working reduced hours or going on short-term disability so that she could focus on her health. We talked about ways for her to get more support for her mother. I also referred her to a social worker in the cancer center so that she would have more help addressing these issues. After every one of our conversations, Julie told me that she still wanted to be positive about her prognosis, and that's great. Talking about your worries doesn't mean that you have to think about them all of the time. Giving them a little airtime allows you to feel less alone and gives you more energy to focus on your health and your immediate goals.

Using the Box

Julie had other concerns about her diagnosis and what the future would look like. It was harder for her to talk about these subjects than it was for her to talk about the practical problems of work and money.

So I introduced her to the idea of the box (also described in chapter 7). I told her that we could tackle one subject at a time, and only for as long as she wanted to talk. She had complete control. She would say, "Let's open the box for a minute." And then she would tell me one of her concerns, which were all of the normal worries. What if the next scan isn't good news? What if I get sick? What if my husband has to care for me? What if that's really hard for him? What if it's too hard for my kids to see me getting worse? What if I die? What will happen to my family?

These concerns were also causing enormous anxiety, and pretending they didn't exist wasn't working for her. We would pick one of these questions and talk about it for as long as she wanted, sometimes only a few minutes. When she felt that we had talked long enough or when she was feeling that the topic was too much, she would say, "I think it's time to close the box." At that point, we would stop. We completely compartmentalized these conversations, and that gave her the confidence to talk about what was bothering her most without the fear of being overwhelmed. Gradually, she was able to make practical plans for what might happen if her cancer got worse and how she and her family could better cope. Eventually she found herself feeling much more like the capable, competent person she had always been.

Medication for Anxiety

Although talking about anxieties can help relieve them, you might have acute episodes of anxiety or panic or ongoing difficulty sleeping that might require medication. In some instances, anxiety feels like a giant wave that can knock you over. Antianxiety medication doesn't take the worries away, but it can help you to keep standing when the wave hits. As with depression, you want to treat anxiety by also making sure that your other symptoms and side effects are under control.

I saw Steve for the first time shortly after his diagnosis with melanoma. At the time he was a theology professor at a local college and a man of strong Christian faith. He had also experienced lifelong struggles with anxiety, but this became much worse when he started what was a particularly difficult course of treatment. Afternoons were the worst for him, and he found that his thoughts raced. The anxiety made him feel awful. Fortunately, he had a good relationship with a therapist, who helped him realize that his diagnosis had caused him to have a crisis of faith. The diagnosis and treatment had shaken many of his beliefs about the world.

In our first appointment, I realized that his physical pain was contributing to his anxiety. He was also taking steroids as part of his chemotherapy regimen, and they were causing anxiety and restlessness. We worked to get his pain under control, which relieved some of his anxiety but not all of it. It became clear that he needed medication to help manage strong generalized anxiety.

Medications such as selective serotonin reuptake inhibitors (SSRIs) can be very helpful for this kind of anxiety. Examples include citalopram (Celexa) or sertraline (Zoloft). Doctors also sometimes prescribe antianxiety medications such as lorazepam (Ativan) for the first two to four weeks, while we are waiting for the SSRI to start working. Sometimes the clinical team worries that combining lorazepam and pain medications can cause confusion. In this situation, I sometimes suggest low doses of a different medication, such as olanzapine (Zyprexa). This kind of medication works more quickly than an SSRI and treats confusion instead of causing it. It is a terrific medication for intense anxiety.

I started Steve on lorazepam and an SSRI, and his anxiety improved a great deal. Now many months later, he has finished all of his treatment, is doing well, and no longer needs either the SSRI or the lorazepam. In his last visit with me, he and his girlfriend both believed that, without treating the anxiety, he wouldn't have been able to get through the chemotherapy treatment that has so effectively treated his cancer.

18

How Does Cancer Affect My Brain?

MANY PEOPLE WORRY THAT THE treatments they receive will affect their thinking. Many patients have heard of "chemo brain," which is a term the medical community has given to the very common complaint from patients that their cognitive function isn't the same when they are taking chemotherapy. Patients will say to me that they feel their thinking isn't as sharp or that they can't complete a brain-teaser or crossword puzzle as easily. They can't multitask the way they used to or concentrate on complicated tasks at work. There are many causes for these complaints, and only sometimes do they involve the chemotherapy. Cancer treatment brings a lot of stressors, including fatigue, anxiety, multiple medications, and a host of medical details to track. Any one of these factors can affect your ability to carry out complex tasks. Radiation to the brain can also cause cognitive impairment.

People are often reluctant to admit to confusion, even to a doctor, but when you do speak up, the doctor can begin to look for some of the known causes and may be able to help. Many times, your doctor will be able to tease out the problem and isolate a medication or other part of treatment that may be contributing to the problem. But doctors take complaints about brain function seriously because once in a while this can indicate that something more urgent is happening. This chapter will describe the most common causes for cognitive impairment and what will happen if the cancer is directly affecting your brain.

What Your Doctor Will Ask

When you are complaining about difficulties with thinking or confusion or your worries about your brain to your clinical team, they are trying to figure out whether it could be caused by the side effects of treatment or whether the cancer itself is directly affecting your brain function. Your medical team will be wondering about a host of possible triggers, and it can take time to sort out all of the possibilities.

I have a patient with stomach cancer that had spread to other organs. Jim is an accountant and his cancer is responding to traditional chemotherapy, but he is noticing that he needs more and more time to complete normal work tasks. He audits several small companies in Boston and can usually finish a preliminary audit within a day. Jim's most recent audit took almost a week. He says it's harder for him to stay on task and he can't remember the details he used to be able to recall easily. To tease out the problem, I asked him all of the questions doctors usually pose in this situation:

- Do you also have headaches?
- Do you have any specific difficulties with movement or walking?
- Do you have difficulty with speaking or seeing things?
- Has anyone ever thought you were confused?
- Do you ever wonder whether you have lost consciousness?
- Has a friend or family member thought that you lost consciousness?

He said no to all of these questions, but I still ordered an MRI to make sure he had no brain metastases. When the MRI came back clear, I sent him to our psychiatric oncologist to make sure that he's not depressed. The doctor told me that Jim has none of the other signs of depression. Many times, doctors will also order a neurological workup to look for specific problems in cognition.

Once we had eliminated the possibility of brain metastases and untreated depression, we could focus on medications that could be causing Jim's problem. After fatigue and stress, medications are the most likely cause of cognitive impairment.

We tried to eliminate his medications one by one to see whether one of them was causing confusion. Sure enough, we found that he was taking lorazepam (Ativan, a benzodiazepine that relieves anxiety) with each chemo session. Jim realized that he was reaching for lorazepam several times per day. This is a drug that can certainly interfere with short-term memory. We limited his lorazepam use to those days when he was receiving chemotherapy, and almost immediately Jim noticed that most but not all of his concentration returned. In some cases, we offer methylphenidate as well to stimulate your ability to concentrate. Methylphenidate is especially helpful with the sedation and cognitive side effects from opioids. We also worked on strategies to help him stay on task and improve his memory, including list-making and cognitive exercises.

Causes of Confusion

Chemotherapy can have some effect on thinking, but there are so many things you go through in treatment that can disrupt your thinking, beyond the chemotherapy drugs themselves:

- Medications, particularly pain medications and benzodiazepines (including antianxiety medications, such as lorazepam). Antinausea meds can also be a culprit.
- Radiation therapy to the brain can cause difficulties in attention, short-term memory, and processing.
- Anxiety and lack of sleep can cause short-term memory difficulties. So can depression.
- Cancer spreading to the brain can cause some of these issues, as well.

Delirium

Some patients experience a temporary but noticeable state of confusion called delirium. It has many potential causes, including something as benign as medication or as easily treatable as a developing infection. But it can also be a sign of a new brain lesion (that is, tumor), a seizure, or a stroke.

I recently admitted one of my colleague's patients to the hospital. Sally has metastatic breast cancer, and her husband became concerned when she woke in the middle of the night and got dressed for work. She seemed to be in a haze, and, when her husband asked her what she was doing, she said, "I have to go to work." He couldn't convince her otherwise. He got dressed and drove her to the hospital, which was the right thing to do.

If a patient experiences delirium, doctors consider this an emergency unless the cause is obvious and reversible. For example, if the patient has taken too much lorazepam or too much of a narcotic, he or she may experience several hours of confusion. Many times the cause isn't obvious, and the patient needs to come to the hospital to go through an evaluation. In the hospital, doctors will take a careful history of events, do a physical exam, and draw blood. The goal is to rule out all the possible causes of delirium. If nothing obvious emerges, doctors usually suggest an MRI and then will consult with neurologists to figure out what's going on.

In Sally's case, the original workup revealed no reason for her confusion. She fell asleep waiting for a bed in the hospital, and when she woke she felt completely normal and showed no signs of confusion. I sat down with her and went over the events of the previous day. Sally remembered dropping her pills on the ground. She thought that she had put all the pills back in their correct bottles but wasn't sure. Her husband produced her pill bottles (it's always good to bring those to the hospital in this kind of emergency). When we looked, we realized that she had mixed up a couple of the pills. As a result, she had taken three times the amount of lorazepam that was prescribed. Because she had tumors in her liver, her body had trouble processing the extra medication, and this had been the cause of her delirium.

Spacing Out

In some cases, delirium or confusion can arise from a more serious cause. My patient Joe had esophageal cancer, and yet he was doing really well on chemotherapy. The cancer had spread to his liver, but treatments were keeping it under control, and he felt well enough to go golfing three times a week and to spend time with his grandchildren. One day he came in for routine chemotherapy, and during our clinic visit I noticed that Joe would space out sometimes. He would stare straight ahead as though he was listening intently but then abruptly reengage with the conversation. At one point I asked him a question, and he didn't answer. Instead, he stared off into the distance. Then he snapped out of it and looked at his wife as though he knew he had missed something. His wife told me that these little episodes had been happening more frequently lately. In the past couple of days, it had become even more noticeable. This isn't technically delirium, but it was affecting his day-to-day life, and I wondered what could be the cause. I ordered an MRI of his brain that afternoon, and it revealed that Joe had multiple brain metastases. These episodes of spacing out had been miniseizures. I got him started right away on antiseizure medication that stopped the episodes and then got him set up for radiation therapy to help treat these metastases.

What If My Cancer Goes to My Brain?

Patients frequently worry about the prospect of their cancer metastasizing to the brain the way that it does to the liver or to any other part of the body. Any cancer can metastasize to the brain, but some cancers have an increased tendency to do this, including breast cancer, lung cancer, and melanoma. Patients who experience the sudden onset of headaches, confusion, or difficulty speaking or moving may be showing signs of brain metastases. Patients who complain of these symptoms will often undergo an MRI of the brain to determine whether this is the case. MRIs are better than CT scans at evaluating the brain.

I worked with a patient who had been diagnosed with stage 4 lung cancer at the age of forty-four. Isaac never smoked and was one of the most physically fit people I have ever met. About a year before I met him, he developed a persistent, dry cough that led to his diagnosis. Molecular pathology showed that he had an ALK translocation (a genetic mutation) that could be treated with the medication crizotinib. The cancer melted away, and Isaac felt so good that he was able to train for and run an Ironman triathlon. Then one day his wife noticed him staring out the window, and she couldn't get his attention for several minutes. When he snapped out of it, he had no recollection of her having spoken to him. She called the clinic, and his oncologist ordered an immediate MRI. I met Isaac as the attending physician on the cancer ward, where I had to tell him that the scan revealed a three-centimeter lesion in his brain that was causing significant swelling, along with three other metastases that were barely visible. His staring episode was a seizure.

Isaac was devastated, as most people are when they first hear that their cancer has spread to the brain. This news can feel overwhelming, but your medical team will put together a plan to address it. Your oncologist will tell you that controlling the disease in the brain will become the primary focus. Sometimes you will be able to continue taking anticancer medication that is controlling the cancer in the rest of your body, but sometimes you will need to put everything on hold, depending on the size, location, and number of metastases involved. Your doctor will also be considering what kind of symptoms you have because of the brain lesions.

Once lesions have been identified, your oncologist will consult with neurosurgeons to see whether they can be removed. Radiation oncologists will also weigh in to determine whether the lesions should be irradiated and if so, how. Sometimes surgeons will want to operate even when they know they can't remove all of the lesions that are causing inflammation in the brain tissue. Remember that the skull is like a wooden box that encases the brain, and it's important to remove whatever cancer we can to relieve the swelling. Doctors might recommend stereotactic radiosurgery (SRS, in which high doses of radiation are delivered to the small area of the cancer nodule), proton beam radiotherapy, or even surgery. In some cases, the whole brain needs to be treated with radiation therapy, which may require that you stop the other anticancer treatments that you are using.

Isaac needed to be admitted to the hospital and to start antiseizure medications, after which his seizures never recurred. Isaac was concerned that he would have to stop the crizotinib, which was controlling his disease, and undergo extensive radiation. Fortunately, in his case, we could continue his targeted therapy, but he would need to undergo extensive radiation to his brain. He was a candidate for SRS to treat the largest of the brain lesions, and his medical team would continue to follow the other nodules with subsequent MRIs. Four months later, I bumped into Isaac in the outpatient clinic, and he told me he had completed his SRS and was continuing to do wonderfully on crizotinib.

If you have brain metastases, your doctor may prescribe steroids such as dexamethasone to keep the swelling at a minimum. Some patients don't like taking steroids, and I can understand why. Over the course of several weeks, steroids can cause your face to swell. You might gain weight, you can develop high blood sugar, and your muscles can weaken. Nevertheless, these drugs can keep your brain functioning well, and sometimes doctors tell patients that they should continue to take them to prevent swelling and inflammation that the brain cancer is causing.

Through a combination of surgery and radiation, doctors can often keep the cancer under control and the brain functioning as normally as possible. One unfortunate limitation of chemotherapy is that it works less well in the brain. Your body is equipped with something called the blood-brain barrier. It works great to keep toxins, including infections, out of your brain even if they are circulating in your system. But this barrier also keeps chemotherapy drugs from circulating in your brain and killing the cancer cells there. That's why someone like Joe can have a great result from chemotherapy in his body, and yet the lesions are freer to grow in his brain.

When treating cancers such as lymphoma of the central nervous system, doctors can bypass the blood-brain barrier and place chemotherapy drugs directly into the cerebrospinal fluid. They do this using a special device, called an Ommaya reservoir, to infuse chemotherapy directly into the brain.

The Role of Rehab

When patients have cancer in the brain, they can sometimes suffer the neurologic damage that is often associated with strokes. They may have balance issues or difficulty speaking and understanding language. When someone has a stroke and is otherwise doing pretty well, doctors suggest physical therapy and occupational therapy as a way to help people regain the skills they may have lost. It's always an option to get these therapies to help you live better and feel better.

In the setting of metastatic cancer, sometimes patients have trouble scheduling these other therapies while receiving intensive treatments for the cancer itself. In some cases, by the time the cancer spreads to the brain, the patient is already exhausted from treatment and from the tumor burden, meaning the amount of cancer in the body. Some patients say to their doctors that they don't really want to spend two to four weeks in a rehab facility practicing walking or learning an exercise regimen because they would rather be at home. Your medical team should understand this request. Your doctors should try to balance this work to regain neurologic function with all of the other demands on you as a patient.

PART III

Dealing with Progressing Cancer

19

They Tell Me the Cancer Is Progressing

IF YOUR CANCER ISN'T CURABLE, there will be a point at which the cancer grows despite chemotherapy and begins to spread. You may decide to read this chapter because scans are showing that the primary tumor has grown or that new tumors have appeared in other parts of your body. If you have been hospitalized for side effects related to the cancer, such as digestive issues or an infection, your doctor may have ordered new scans to see whether these have been caused by the spread of cancer. In some cases, patients have had a great response from targeted therapies or standard chemotherapy, and then suddenly they become ill with a complication from the cancer.

When your doctor says that the cancer is progressing despite treatment, then he or she is telling you that you are at a different phase of treatment. This can be hard to accept. Many patients tell me that they needed weeks or even months to understand fully that their cancer was advancing. Patients often ask me what it means to have advancing cancer. I say that up to now your medical team has been working to minimize the symptoms and side effects of treatment, but in the future we will be working with you to minimize the side effects of the cancer itself. This may involve more interventions to prevent tumors from interfering with your digestion or your breathing, and to prevent bleeding issues and future infections. You may also need more help minimizing pain. Not everyone will have these symptoms. Some people have few side effects of advancing cancer except for an increase in fatigue and weight loss.

At this point your doctor may also talk to you about the possibility of enrolling in a clinical trial to help evaluate new drugs to treat your type of cancer.

Entering a New Phase

Hearing that you are in a new phase of treatment can make you feel vulnerable all over again. Many patients say that learning that the primary tumor is growing or that new metastases have become visible is a shock similar to the one they felt when they were first diagnosed. In the next chapter, Vicki will talk about how to cope in this new phase, how to develop a good awareness of the likely course and outcome of your disease, and what to hope for when you can't hope for a cure. Getting oriented in this new reality takes time, and you need to be patient with yourself.

This is the phase of treatment in which your oncologist is going to be paying even more attention to symptoms and side effects of the cancer itself, even though you may be switching to a new line of chemotherapy.

One of my recent patients had a particularly difficult time with this. Janine was a teacher in her late fifties with pancreatic cancer, and she had responded extremely well to the first line of chemotherapy. She was on it for about eighteen months and felt great. Then the cancer became resistant, and she needed to switch to a second line of treatment. I explained that we were in a different phase of treatment, in which the cancer would be harder to control, and Janine told me that she understood. Then a few weeks later, she came into the clinic complaining of abdominal discomfort. I told Janine that I wanted to start her on some pain medication, and she seemed shocked. She told me that the tumors would shrink again now that she had started the new drug because that is what had happened with her first line of chemotherapy. Of course, I hoped that this would be true and that she would have a great response to this second line of treatment. But, as her oncologist, I also worried about what would happen if the treatment didn't work as well as we both hoped. I wanted her to understand that we had to stay on top of new side effects so that she wouldn't struggle with them in the next six months. In retrospect, I realized that this was the first time Janine really began to understand that her cancer was incurable.

A second line of chemo is usually second because research shows that it is less likely to control the cancer in most patients than the first line. The same is true for a third line. It's at this point in treatment that your oncologist is starting to get worried about chemotherapy's ability to control your cancer. Every cancer is a bit different, and some patients can get a good response to second and third line chemotherapy. However, sometimes the cancer doesn't respond the way we are hoping it will. Remember that you didn't fail the chemotherapy. People like to think that they somehow control the good responses, through diet or exercise or supplements or meditation. If they believe that logic, then when a new line of chemotherapy doesn't work, they believe that they didn't do something correctly. Cancer is biological just like an infection. If you had a urinary tract infection, and it stopped responding to a particular antibiotic, you would try a new antibiotic. We do the same thing in cancer treatment. If the new drug doesn't work as well as the last one, there is a biological explanation. Your tumor is resistant to the biological pathway that a particular chemotherapy uses to attack the cancer cells.

Resistance to Targeted Therapy

Not everyone enters this phase after undergoing chemotherapy. Some patients have been taking targeted therapies for months or years with extraordinary results before the cancer becomes resistant. Vicki worked with a patient who had lung cancer even though she had never smoked. Nancy's cancer had been caused by a genetic mutation—called an ALK mutation—that was highly responsive to crizotinib, which she took in pill form. She had no infusions and came to the clinic once a month to check in. She felt terrific for three years, and then one day came in with headaches and a drooping eye-lid. An MRI of her brain revealed that little clumps of tumor had begun to grow on the lining covering her brain. She had some radia-tion and started chemotherapy, but it wasn't as effective. It was a heartbreaking transition for Nancy to go from feeling nearly normal to having brain metastases that were hard to treat. She told Vicki that it was like being diagnosed all over again.

I have seen patients like this as well. Tom was a sixty-one-year-old construction worker with esophageal cancer. He was fortunate in that his cancer cells had an abnormality of the HER2 gene, so we were able to start him on a combination of standard chemotherapy with a drug that attacked the HER2 pathway. The tumors through-out his body melted away, including the lesions (tumors) in his liver. Tom was acutely aware that he wasn't like the other patients with esophageal cancer in the infusion unit. The friends he made there didn't do as well as he did, and he often told me how lucky he was to be on a targeted therapy. One day he came into the clinic complaining of abdominal discomfort. He wanted to know whether it was consti-pation. But his pain didn't seem consistent with constipation, and, in fact, it was caused by small tumors in the liver. His cancer had grown through the chemotherapy and become resistant to the tar-geted therapy. I told Tom that we would have to switch him to a second line of chemotherapy or enroll him in a clinical trial that was testing a new drug. He seemed incredulous and asked why there wasn't another HER2 targeted therapy. I had to explain that we are in a new era of targeted therapies, and treatments are still being developed. Entering this new phase of treatment is difficult for everyone, but I think it can be especially disorienting for people who have had a fantastic and sustained response to the first line of treatment.

Best- and Worst-Case Scenarios

This is a good time to ask your oncologist to give you an idea about the best- and worst-case scenarios for this new line of treatment. The situation has changed because the cancer has become resistant to one or more drugs, and you will want to get a picture of what the future might hold at this time. There is still a lot of uncertainty, but this might be a time when the best-case scenario is measured in months rather than years.

Sometimes when a patient changes to a new line of therapy, he or she may feel sicker from the cancer or because the body has already endured a lot of infusions. This can be a tough time for some patients because they feel their body isn't tolerating the infusions or the medications in the same way. Other patients do well even though their cancer is still slowly growing through the chemotherapy. It is different for everyone. Your oncologist can't predict how you will respond to this new line.

Whenever you switch to a new line of chemotherapy, your doctor will review with you the likely side effects of the new drugs. He or she should also let you know that more chemotherapy isn't always better and that there may come a time when chemotherapy treatments can shorten your life rather than extend it.

Symptom Management

At this time, your medical team members should be asking you a lot of questions about how you feel physically. They will be paying particular attention to your blood counts and to pain and fatigue, and they will review with you the signs of infection and the signs of any bleeding issues. This is the time to pick up the phone and call the clinic or your doctor if anything seems off or if you are struggling to manage your symptoms at home. Your oncologist and nurse practitioner want to work actively with you to adjust any medications and keep you feeling your best. I always ask people how they are sleeping, what they do during the day, and how their bodies respond to the infusions.

Vicki and I have reviewed the major symptoms in the previous ten chapters, and these will help guide you through any new issues that arise at this time. As cancer progresses, we pay particular attention to pain management, any difficulty eating, the possibility of bone marrow failure, and fatigue.

Pain Management

Some patients notice a change in the intensity of pain as their cancer progresses. Cancer can spread to the bones, or it can spread to abdominal organs and tissues, which might make it more difficult to move or sleep comfortably. Even if you have avoided pain medication to this point, your doctor might encourage you to manage your pain actively. If you have been taking pain medication, your doctor will be asking whether it's still working. We worry at this time about opioid tolerance and about intractable pain, which means pain that's not responding to opioids.

Tolerance to Opioids

Patients who have taken opioids for pain for some time may have noticed that the doses have increased over time. That's normal and expected as long as the pain can be managed by higher doses. If at some point you are taking long-acting opioids and still need several doses of short-acting pain medication to handle breakthrough pain, your doctor may wonder whether you have developed some tolerance for the opioids you are taking. This means that your brain has increased the number of receptors for that specific kind of opioid. Patients sometimes experience this if they have slow-growing tumors and have been in treatment for several years. The usual fix is to increase the dose or try a different pain medication. Doctors call the process of switching drugs opioid rotation.

One patient at the clinic, Jill, had a slow-growing breast cancer that had spread to her bones. She was doing great with antiestrogen therapy. Her tumor markers (levels of proteins secreted by cancer cells; see chapter 6) remained low, and her CT scans showed stable disease. Despite the stability of the cancer, her bone pain increased over a period of two months. With her oncologist's guidance, she tried increasing her oxycodone for immediate pain relief. Then they increased her Oxycontin, her long-acting medication. The pain would respond for a couple of days to these newer doses and then return. Her doctor switched her to a different medication, in this case a fentanyl patch, to help with ongoing pain, and gave her Dilaudid for those times when the pain increased sharply. Within one week, she was back to baseline with her pain.

When you change your opioid medication, you will have to work closely with your oncologist or palliative care specialist. There will be some experimentation to find the right dose of the new medication. Sometimes I ask patients to be admitted to the hospital to do this because we can give IV medications while the nurses are supervising you. We can find the appropriate dose much more quickly that way.

Treatments for Intractable Pain

In those cases where pain management becomes an ongoing issue, we sometimes think of using intravenous medications instead of oral narcotics or pain patches. This doesn't mean staying in the hospital hooked up to an IV. Patients can use something called patient-controlled analgesia (PCA), which is a pump often used by people recovering from surgery. It comes with a button you can push to deliver more pain medication as needed. This is a wonderful tool that gives people a sense of control over their own medication while living at home.

Another option is something called intrathecal pain medication, which is sort of like having an epidural during childbirth. The pain specialist will insert a tiny catheter into the spine in an area that will give the patient the most relief. Then he or she will fill a pump that is also implanted inside the body. The benefit is that the pump sends pain medication, such as an opioid, directly at the affected nerves and keeps them from sending pain signals to the brain. As a result, you can reduce the level of opioid pain medication and the side effects that come with them. The downside is that it's cumbersome to use. A pain specialist has to refill the pump, and, because it's inside your body, it can become a source for infection. Doctors tend to recommend this option when escalating doses of oral or IV medications don't provide relief or come with intolerable side effects.

Always remember that radiation to a particular location of cancer can result in dramatic improvements in pain control. This is particularly useful for cancers that are in the bone or cancers that are pressing against a nerve.

Difficulty Eating

As the cancer progresses, it creates new tumors in different areas of the body, and existing tumors grow. Eventually tumors may appear in the digestive tract, or they may encroach on the stomach or a section of the intestines, making eating or digesting food more difficult. If this happens, you may notice an increase in abdominal cramps, nausea, or constipation for which the usual medications don't seem to work. Your doctors are going to continue to ask about bowel movements, about your nausea, and about your food and water intake. Your doctor may press on your abdomen to check for distention.

If your doctor suspects a gastrointestinal (GI) obstruction, he or she will probably order a CT scan to look at the digestive tract. There are several possible solutions to relieve the discomfort and get things moving again.

Surgery. A surgeon might be able to bypass an obstruction in the intestines by looping a section of the intestine around the tumor. You should know that the surgeon will probably not remove the tumor itself because that kind of surgery is much more invasive and the risks of complications may be too high. Looping the bowel around an obstruction, which is called a bypass operation, can be highly effective at getting people back to eating and digesting food, but not everyone is a good candidate for surgery. Sometimes the tumor is located in a spot that surgeons can't easily reach. Sometimes the extent of cancer in the abdomen makes surgery tricky or unlikely to succeed. If surgery is not an option, your doctor may suggest other techniques for relieving the obstruction.

Radiation. Your doctor may suggest radiation treatments to reduce tumors obstructing the upper GI tract (the esophagus, stomach, or duodenum) or tumors in the lowest part of the GI tract (the rectum or anal canal). While these treatments often work effectively to relieve an obstruction, they don't work as quickly as surgery. You may need several weeks of radiation treatments to see results, and this can be difficult to tolerate in the short term.

Enteral Stents. If radiation isn't an option, your doctor may suggest inserting a metal tube, or stent, which is a lot like the coronary stents used to prop open arteries. The obvious drawback with stents is that they aren't as elastic as the natural bowel. With an enteral stent, you may have to restrict the amount of food you take in at any one time. They can also clog easily, so you may be put on a liquid or pureed diet if you have a stent in the stomach or upper GI tract, and if you have a stent in the rectum or anal canal, you may have to take extra laxatives to keep the stool soft enough to pass through the stent easily.

Venting G-Tube. If nothing else works, surgeons may need to find a way to drain accumulating fluids from the GI tract. A surgeon or interventional radiologist can insert a tube through the upper abdomen and into the stomach. This allows patients to drain fluid from the stomach whenever they feel nausea, so they can feel as though they can keep liquids and nutrients down, even if they can't pass through the rest of the intestinal tract. The downside is that patients with a G-tube can't take in solid foods anymore because they will clog the tube.

Bone Marrow Failure

Chemotherapy is hard on your bone marrow. All along you've had blood tests to measure your body's ability to make healthy blood cells. At some point you may find that the cancer or treatment has wiped out your bone marrow. This makes you more susceptible to infection and bleeding, which your doctor will work to control.

Patients with hematologic malignancies (cancers of the blood; see chapter 4) are most susceptible to bone marrow failure, particularly those with myelodysplastic syndrome, chronic leukemia, lymphoma, and multiple myeloma. But some solid cancers such as breast cancer and melanoma eventually cause bone marrow failure when the cancer cells spread to the bone marrow enough to displace the normal blood cells growing there.

You will know whether your doctor is worried about bone marrow failure because your blood tests will indicate low levels of red cells, white cells, and platelets. Many things can cause low blood counts, so you don't have to immediately worry that your bone marrow is failing if your blood counts are low. But when all three types of cells are low, a condition called pancytopenia, we begin to worry that cancer cells are filling up the bone marrow. In this case, your doctor may order a bone marrow biopsy. This sometimes shows the cancer cells spread out in sheets across the bone marrow and the absence of hematopoiesis, which is the development of new blood cells. The process of cancer spread inside the bone marrow is also called myelophthisis. Having low blood counts leaves patients more prone to several conditions. They may have bleeding issues because of low platelets, infections from low white cells, and heart disease from low red blood cells.

In chapter 15, on bleeding issues, I described transfusions of both red blood cells and platelets as a treatment for low blood counts. While this is effective with red cells and platelets, we don't transfuse white blood cells because they will attack normal cells. Also, continuing to receive frequent transfusions can be problematic because patients can develop allergies to the different components in transfused blood. Your medical team will continue to try to manage these low counts in whatever way they can, which may mean several transfusions, if these are deemed safe.

Fatigue

Most people experience increased fatigue after their cancer stops responding to treatment. Early on in treatment, you may have experienced fatigue from the chemotherapy or radiation treatments, but you bounced back after a few days. As the cancer spreads, you may have to ration your energy more carefully.

Jose was a longstanding parish priest whom I took care of for several years. He had metastatic colon cancer and initially did remarkably well with chemotherapy. He had no pain, no nausea, no shortness of breath. He would receive letters every day from people he had married or had ministered to over the years, and keeping up that correspondence was something he greatly enjoyed. As his cancer progressed, he struggled with writing even a paragraph. Jose told me that he had prepared to suffer from his cancer with pain or nausea but that he never quite realized the suffering that would come from fatigue. It physically pained him that he was too tired to interact with people on a regular basis. Unfortunately, fatigue caused by cancer is very hard to control. If you can't control it, you have to work around it. Vicki often tells people to take note of those times of day when they feel most energetic and plan to do important tasks during those times. Save your energy for those things that matter most.

Treatment Options

This is a time when patients and families ask about alternative therapies. Some take a new interest in nutritional supplements, which Vicki discussed in chapter 13. Others wonder about experimental drugs in other countries and ask whether there isn't something else to try. Or they ask about expensive overseas clinics that mix alternative therapies with standard care. (In chapter 22, I will explain why I advise against this.)

New experimental drugs are being tested all the time, and the best way to get access to them is to enroll in a clinical trial. But a clinical trial isn't for everyone. For some, it means traveling to a clinical research center, which may be expensive or inconvenient. Others have an immediate aversion to this idea. They don't want to take drugs that are still being tested. They don't want to be Chuck Yeager flying a new kind of airplane. They want only standard, proven treatments, and that's great. A clinical trial is just an option. But sometimes participating in a clinical trial is the only way to access new treatments for your disease.

Clinical Trials

At this point, you might ask your doctor about the possibility of participating in a clinical trial. Before you decide, you should know how clinical trials work and what each phase of a trial hopes to accomplish.

Phase I. This is sometimes called a first-in-human study. Researchers who have tested a promising new treatment in the lab need to find out whether it is tolerable in humans and at what dose it might be effective. Phase I trials typically enroll patients with advanced cancers for whom the standard treatments are no longer working.

Phase II. These typically enroll between thirty and fifty patients who will receive the same dose and schedule of a new drug that has completed phase I testing. In this phase, doctors are still testing the safety of a new drug, but they will also measure how effectively it either shrinks the cancer or keeps it stable. We call this the response rate. It's always good to ask the physicians running the trial what they would consider a success in this clinical trial. This will give you a good idea of what to expect.

Phase III. These are randomized trials, meaning that you will be randomly enrolled in one of two arms, or groups of patients, of the study. A computer assigns you to receive either standard care alone or standard care plus the new drug. You don't get to choose which arm of the study you will join, but you will usually know whether you are receiving the new treatment or not, and so will your doctors. At this point, researchers are comparing the efficacy of the new treatment to standard care. A few studies contain a placebo arm, meaning neither the patient nor the doctor knows whether you are taking the new drug or getting standard care. Many placebo arm studies take place outside the United States.

You don't need to be frightened by clinical trials. Instead, you can ask your oncologist which studies are going on for patients with your type of cancer. This should prompt a good discussion about the current standard of care and what kind of drugs are emerging for your type of cancer.

While enrolling in a clinical trial can be an appropriate option at any point, it tends to be more of an option as cancer worsens. You don't have to be treated at a teaching hospital to participate in one of these studies. Clinical research takes place in many nonacademic settings.

Informed Consent

Many people agonize over the decision to enroll in a study. Before you consent, your oncologist will explain what the study is and describe what's known about the new drug. He or she will tell you about the possibility of toxicity and also describe exactly what the study will measure. In some cases, researchers are hoping to extend life expectancy for just a few extra months, or they are hoping for a response rate that is slightly higher than that of standard care. For some people, this is a difficult conversation because it highlights the fact that their cancer has progressed to the point where standard care can't control it anymore and that even the newest treatments won't bring a cure.

I remember conducting one of these conversations early in my career. Hazel was a sixty-eight-year-old woman with metastatic breast cancer who was trying to decide whether to enroll in a clinical trial I was running for a new chemotherapy drug. Her cancer had grown through the first line of treatment, and she seemed very interested in the idea of receiving a new drug. I explained to her in technical terms what we were hoping to measure in the study: we were hoping for a response rate that was 30 percent instead of 20 percent, and we were hoping to extend progression-free survival by two to three months. She smiled at me and said that she was hoping for a cure. I smiled back at her and explained again what the study would measure. We did this exchange a couple of times before Hazel stopped me and said, "You think I didn't hear you the first time?" She said, "I'm allowed to hope and you're not allowed to take that away from me." She was right. I thought she wasn't listening to me. Instead, I was the one not listening to her.

In this discussion, you can and should ask a lot of questions about the study and how it will be conducted, and what life is like in a clinical trial. If you do enroll, you should know that your life will be busier than it is in standard care. You will meet regularly with a clinical research nurse who is responsible for the conduct of the trial and who will make sure that the oncologist is doing everything exactly as the protocols dictate. You may have extra blood tests to document how quickly the drug clears out of your system (called pharmacokinetics) and extra scans and other tests to determine how the drug is affecting your body (called pharmacodynamics). Behind the scenes, a clinical research coordinator will collect all the data from your tests and scans and document in exhaustive detail your progress throughout the trial. He or she will also make sure that regulatory documents have been filled out.

Before you can enroll, the oncologist will have to get your informed consent. This entails a long discussion about every aspect of the trial and everything that will be expected of you, and you will need to sign a document stating that you understand everything about the study and the risks involved. You should have a good understanding of all of these facts before you sign a consent document. You should also understand that you can withdraw your consent at any time during the study without fear of any repercussions. This is one of the first principles of medical ethics when it comes to clinical trials.

Family Meetings

Some people try to hide the news that the cancer is progressing from family and close friends, telling themselves that they don't want to burden anyone. Countless patients have told me that they will tell their adult children about this later, at some future point, but that point never seems to come. And then I get phone calls from these close family members demanding to know what's going on. They are often in tears, and they feel hurt or betrayed by the patient's silence. By law, I cannot disclose information about a patient to anyone without the patient's permission. So, at this point, I often suggest a family meeting, which is a chance for the patient, the medical team members, and key family members to sit in the same room and discuss the treatment plan.

You can request a family meeting at any time, but these can be especially powerful when your treatment options are changing or when the cancer is beginning to grow through the chemotherapy. Your doctor can help you break the news to family members and talk in concrete terms about next steps. Your doctor can lay out the best-case scenario and the worst-case scenario, just as he or she did when you were first diagnosed. For patients, this is a chance to say to everyone what you want and don't want in terms of treatment and for everyone to hear your wishes. It's easy to believe that information will worry people, but the truth is that your family already feels concerned about what is happening and about what might happen next, and silence only makes their anxiety worse.

20

Living and Hoping
with Advancing Cancer

I OFTEN MEET WITH PATIENTS for the first time after they have been told that their cancer is incurable or that it has begun to grow through treatment. They have worked hard to become capable cancer patients. Most of them have figured out a system for dealing with the side effects of treatment and have continued to work or volunteer. Perhaps they have gone on trips and spent extra time with their families. They have lived as normally as possible for many months or several years. And they have focused on everything the oncologist has focused on, which is getting through treatments with the hope that the cancer will continue to be held in check.

It's disorienting to be told that treatments are no longer keeping the cancer from spreading, even when you have been through multiple lines of chemotherapy, even when you have had a health crisis that shows the spread of tumors (metastases) to new areas of the body, even when you feel a lot of fatigue. It's difficult to understand what might happen next, no matter how much you know about your diagnosis.

For example, I worked closely with Terry, who was diagnosed with stage 4 ovarian cancer at the age of fifty-two. Although she had made her living as a nurse and understood the staging of cancer, she told her oncologist that she refused to think about the fact that she might die. Fortunately, she responded very well to chemotherapy for several years. She had been in treatment for more than three years by the time I met her. After her first line of chemo stopped working, and then the second line, she got frustrated with her oncologist. The truth was that she had trouble believing that the cancer was getting worse, even though she had multiple tumors in her abdomen and liver and was struggling to manage her fatigue enough to go to work. Terry was a smart, dedicated medical professional, and yet she needed help understanding what was happening in her body. A lot of people do.

In this chapter, I'm going to describe some strategies you can use to cope with this confusion and the anxiety that comes with it. In palliative care we talk about a concept called prognostic awareness, and I'll explain what that is. But we also talk a lot about hope—and what to hope for in this challenging time. You can continue to hope and to make plans, even if you aren't hoping for a cure.

What Is Prognostic Awareness?

At many points after diagnosis, people wonder whether they might die from cancer. Early on in treatment, it's easier to push these thoughts away and pretend they don't exist. Sometimes they pop up again when you are awake at 3 a.m. or when you are alone and feeling down. Even when these thoughts become consuming, most people don't share them with anyone. It can feel disloyal to talk about the possibility of death with people who are working to support you while you are going through treatment.

During my first appointment with Terry, we talked about a lot of subjects, including pain management, fatigue, and finding some ways for her to continue to work as a nurse, which she really loved. Then I asked her what she hoped for and what she was worried about. For some people, this is the first time anyone has asked this question and actually wanted to hear the answer.

"I'm terrified that I might die from this," she said. Terry believed that optimism was the only thing that was keeping her cancer in check. She was afraid that she would be letting her family and friends down if she admitted that she had moments of real sadness. Although she told her family and her doctor that she was going to beat this, she actually worried constantly about the cancer getting worse.

In fact, Terry was afraid that saying anything out loud about dying was inviting her cancer to get worse. But there is no data to suggest that this is true. Talking about it doesn't make it happen. In fact, all the energy you exert trying not to think about it or talk about it can be exhausting. You should not be going through this alone.

The process of understanding your illness is called prognostic awareness, and it takes time to develop. You don't have to make sense of all of this difficult information about the future all at once. You can and should do it in stages. The first stage is having a conversation about what you hope for and what you worry about. Over many subsequent conversations with Terry, I asked her to think about and talk about what might happen. What if the disease got worse? What would that mean, and what decisions would we need to think about together? What if she had to stop working? What if she was hospitalized? Talking about these issues doesn't mean they are going to happen. But it's vital to have some safe place to think out loud and to create a possible plan B. Your care team can help you start these conversations.

There is a lot of uncertainty with serious cancer. Things can change slowly over time, or they might change quickly. Most people need at least some sense of the future to inform their decisions about future treatments. That's why having some prognostic awareness, some ability to talk about the future, is so critical.

Am I in Denial?

I also remind patients that they don't have to have prognostic awareness all the time. In palliative care, we think of this awareness as a pendulum that swings back and forth. One minute you think you've got a handle on it, and then the next minute you feel certain that the diagnosis is a big mistake and that the doctors are just wrong.

Patients sometimes ask me, "Am I in denial? Sometimes I just pretend that things are fine. I know that what we talk about is true, but I just don't want to think about it all the time." This is perfectly normal. It is impossible to live with a constant awareness that time is shorter than you had hoped. Few patients are completely in denial. And no matter how much prognostic awareness you have, there's still room to hope for a miracle.

I recently interviewed a doctor at Mass General, a patient of Dave's, who had serious cancer and was about to go home to hospice care. I wanted to videotape our conversation so that a group of medical trainees could learn more about what it's like to live with a serious illness. I knew Doug would be the perfect person to talk to young doctors about how it feels to go through this. I asked Doug what he expected for the future. He said, "I know we have to wait and see. I know it might be months. It might be weeks. I'm going to go home with hospice, but I sort of want to believe that there's a 5 percent chance that Dave is going to walk in here and say he's found the perfect thing for me."

Doug didn't feel this way because he lacked awareness about his illness. He felt it because he is human. The truth is that Dave and I wished the same thing too. It is normal to understand and then forget. Making sense of all of this all at once is impossible.

Later on, Doug said something in the interview that will stay with me forever. He was addressing the young medical students that he knew would watch the video. "I have no regrets," he said. "Listen guys, we all get to go to the party. And it's our job to make that party as good as we can make it. We don't all get to leave the party at the same time. Some of us have to leave the party early. But that doesn't mean it wasn't a damn good party."

Am I Giving Up Hope?

Some people are reluctant to talk at all about the possibility of death. Families sometimes worry that having these conversations might make the patient depressed or give up on treatment. Patients also worry that, once they acknowledge the possibility of dying, then they will have to experience all of the feelings that come with that possibility all at once. Or they worry that they will have to immediately solve all of the logistical concerns and family concerns that come with that possibility. And so people tell themselves that talking about death in any context is the same thing as giving up hope.

Becoming more comfortable with the idea that this cancer may take your life someday is not giving up hope. On the contrary, denying a difficult truth can be exhausting and stressful. I helped to conduct an early intervention palliative care study to see how patients reacted when asked to talk about these issues in a manner that was not overwhelming. The study showed that the people who had a place to voice their concerns slowly over time had a better quality of life, a 50 percent lower rate of depression, and lived longer than those who were not receiving early palliative care in which they were able to talk about death.

Won't My Oncologist Bring It Up?

Some clinicians are reluctant to bring up the subject of death with patients. And research shows that doctors and their patients sometimes collude to avoid these conversations. Remember that your clinical team is made up of professionals who also get attached to their patients. The doctors and nurses in oncology work so closely with patients and their families. The oncologists I've worked with truly love their patients and fervently hope that treatments will work. Giving the news that treatment isn't working anymore is really hard for them, too. While many of them are comfortable initiating conversations about the next phase of the illness, a few of them wait for patients to initiate these conversations.

If you want more information about the likely future with your illness, raise these questions with your care team. You can ask many of the same questions I asked Terry. What might happen next? What if the cancer gets worse? What would that be like? How long do people with my type of cancer usually live after the treatment stops working?

How Much Do I Want to Know?

I always ask people to think about what kind of information would be helpful to know and when. There are no right or wrong answers.

I've found that people think very differently about medical treatments if they have years to live rather than months or weeks. With more knowledge, they can make practical plans such as whether to take a vacation or change the date of a family event to make more certain that they can attend. Or they want to know specifically whether they are likely to be alive for a major holiday or life event, such as a child or grandchild's graduation.

Other people are less interested in how much time they might have and instead want to know more about how they might feel as the illness progresses. Will I have more fatigue? Will I be able to work much longer? How much support will I need at home?

How Much Time Do I Have?

If you do ask your doctor to tell you how long you might live, be aware that no doctor can be completely certain about this. Typically, doctors think is in terms of a range of possible outcomes, perhaps measured in years, months, or weeks. Another way that clinicians talk about the future is in terms of best-case, worst-case, and most likely scenarios. Sometimes the best-case scenario is also the most likely, but sometimes it isn't.

I like to tell patients what I am hoping for and what I am worried about. A patient of mine, Tom, was about to go home to hospice care. He was quite ill from his cancer. He asked me how long I thought he had. At the time, I was worried it could be as short as a few weeks. I told him I hoped that I was wrong and that it was more like months. As it turns out, he had a delayed response to chemotherapy and the tumors stopped growing. We disenrolled him from hospice so that he could start a new treatment regimen, and he lived another nine months. When he came back to see me at the clinic for help with his pain management, I asked him how he felt about my inaccurate estimate. He smiled. "You said you hoped you would be wrong and you were. I figured you were just really happy that you were wrong," he said. It's true. I was so happy to be wrong. Tom wasn't disappointed. He found that having the information that his time might be quite short helped him to prepare his family.

It is the fear of being inaccurate that keeps so many clinicians from these discussions about time. I find that most people just want to know in broad terms what their doctor thinks is likely. They don't hold us to it, but it gives them a range that is helpful.

Sometimes you ask for information about how long you might live and then struggle to remember what was said. It can be difficult to process this information the first time you hear it. I had a patient named Gene who had liver cancer at the age of fifty-eight. Gene was able to get a liver transplant and did well after surgery. Unfortunately, he was then diagnosed with esophageal cancer. Gene and I met with his oncologist, and at this meeting Gene asked whether he would be alive for Christmas, which was in three months. His oncologist said that Christmas was a stretch, but that he had a good shot of making it to his birthday, which was in one month.

Later that day, Gene told his oncology fellow that the senior oncologist had told him that he had between six and eight months to live. Then when Gene's wife came to see him, Gene told her that he didn't know what the future would hold and that he just wanted to take things in two-week increments. Was Gene in denial all day? Probably not. He was slowly acclimating to a very difficult reality. Integrating information like this takes time, and not everyone can hear a piece of information like this and hang onto it.

Can I Change My Mind?

It's also perfectly okay to change your mind and to want more information at one point and less later on. I worked with a patient named Diane who was in her seventies and living with ovarian cancer. She would sometimes ask me a question about the future and then stop herself, saying, "On second thought. I don't want to know." She told me that the cancer is what it is and that she and her family would have to figure things out as they happened. I knew that Diane had good prognostic awareness. She wasn't refusing to talk about the future because she thought the doctors were wrong or because she thought that she would still be cured. Instead, she knew that having a lot of information about different potential developments wouldn't be helpful for her in her goal of living her life fully. She wanted to focus on the activities that she could still do that she still loved to do.

About a year later, Diane was hospitalized with an obstruction in her bowels, and she asked me to tell her exactly how long I thought she had to live and what that time might be like. I asked her why she wanted this information because she had been so adamant about not talking about it before. Diane told me that she worried that her children didn't understand how sick she was. "I feel that I need to know more now so that I can tell them," she said. So we had a long conversation about the likely trajectory of her illness, and she shared that information with her children. She wanted to know whether she had weeks or months to live so that she could make plans and help her children prepare.

In our most recent visits, Diane has told me that she wants to go back to not talking about the future. She has even told her oncologist that she doesn't want to know the results of her CT scans. "We are where we are," she said to me. "What good does it do me?"

There are times when the person living with cancer wants more or less information than the family wants. You can probably work out a plan where the doctor will have a slightly different conversation with you than he or she has when family are present. Sometimes people living with cancer want to take things as they come, while family members want more detailed information about what might happen next so they can plan for hospice care or family leave. Sometimes the patient really wants to know all the available information about the future, but the family doesn't. Sometimes the patient doesn't want to have any sort of timeline about the future, but the family really wants to know in order to prepare. I usually ask both the patient and the loved ones what information would be helpful and defer to the patient's preferences. Sometimes the patient asks that I talk with the family, but they don't want to know. That is fine with me as long as the patient is okay with it.

Coping without Getting Down

As my patients begin to hold a deeper understanding of the likely illness trajectory, it can be hard to know how to cope effectively and stay focused on living fully. It doesn't help when other people spout annoying platitudes because they don't know what else to say. Some people tell my patients simplistic things, such as, "Live each day to the fullest!" One of my patients had this sarcastic reply: "Sure. I'll get right on that." Another patient said, "Seriously? Why don't you try it sometime?"

The truth is that people with advancing cancer are living with a foot in two worlds. They live in the world with their family and friends where they want to make plans and accomplish goals. But they also live in a world where they have a sense that life is going to be different from what they'd hoped for. This is a sad, often painful, reality.

I remind people at this time that feeling down is normal. One of my patients insisted to me that she was depressed and told me that she was sobbing the day before because she could no longer take her long daily walks. Her neuropathy had become so bad that she could no longer play her favorite pieces on the piano. The cancer was taking things away from her that she really loved to do. When I asked her how she spent her time, she told me that she visits her grandchildren every chance she gets. They watch silly movies together and play games. She spends time with her friends. I had to tell her that just because you are sad doesn't mean you are depressed. She was clearly able to find joy in life, and it was okay for her to feel sad about what she could no longer do.

My patients tell me that it is most helpful if they give themselves and their family members permission to just forget about the illness at times. When they do talk to loved ones about difficult subjects, they limit those conversations and give cues about when they are ready to talk about something serious. When they've had enough, they say so. And that gives everyone the signal that it's time to talk about other matters and maybe forget about the illness if they can.

People who cope especially well at this time are the people who keep making plans that help them look forward to something in the future. I always ask people what they are looking forward to. It might be a visit to see family or a walk on the beach. It could be anything, such as a tour of major ballparks, a woodworking project, a hobby you have hoped to engage in more fully. Now is the time. It is critical to keep a forward momentum.

Having a practice of gratitude can also be helpful. Even in the midst of something as difficult as cancer, people can develop an appreciation for this new perspective on life. Some people start to think in terms of gratitude for those they love and their work and their spiritual community. Instead of thinking solely about all that they have lost to the cancer, they try to notice everything they have, including the support of good friends, work they love, their spiritual life, or even a devoted pet. My patients tell me that focusing on what they have and what they love is a powerful antidote for the feeling that cancer is running their lives.

Some of my patients do something that I still find amazing. They express gratitude for aspects of their illness. One patient, Joe, recently said to me, "I would never have asked for this. Never. But I can't deny that everything is different for me. I love my wife more. I could just sit and watch my kids play for hours. This spring when the blossoms came out on the trees, I saw how magnificent they were. I'd never appreciated that before. I know it sounds corny, but I don't take things for granted the way I used to."

Joe is unusual. Having cancer doesn't automatically make you appreciate everything more, and you don't have to try to do that if it's not your style. People like Joe understand the burdens of cancer. They know how much treatment has encroached on their autonomy. But they can still stay curious about how this new perspective has changed their relationships, and through this curiosity they are better able to partner with the cancer. They don't have to think of it solely as an enemy, and they don't have to think in terms of winning or losing a battle. They look for ways to say, "I'm still me. This is still my life."

21

What about Practical Concerns?

SOME PEOPLE WILL HAVE AN ONCOLOGIST say to them that they need to get their affairs in order. It can be hard to figure out exactly what that means beyond meeting with an accountant, if appropriate, or having a current will. You may want to create a spreadsheet with account numbers for insurance policies and passwords for e-mail accounts and bank accounts, and you may want to communicate your wishes for any funeral arrangements. These discussions with family members can be fraught with anxiety because the people who love and support you may say they prefer to not talk about these things. But I've found that these same family members will have an easier time later on if you've been firm with them about making arrangements while you still feel well enough to organize these details.

Think of this chapter as a way of taking some unpleasant medicine that will make things better, even though you may have to figure out how to get it down. When you have a serious illness like cancer, there is some really basic planning that you can get out of the way, knowing you will feel better afterward.

Choosing a Health Care Proxy

It's important to have someone assigned to make medical decisions for you if necessary. This may be called a health care proxy or a durable power of attorney for health care. It's a legal document that you have to sign, and in some states you need an attorney to draw up the forms. In some states, you can download a form and fill it out as long as witnesses sign with you.

When you choose someone to act as a health care proxy agent, make sure this person knows you well and will be able to make decisions as you would. You want to choose someone who lives near you and can travel easily to a hospital to make these decisions and someone who will be a strong advocate for your wishes even in the presence of conflicting opinions from family members or friends.

Have a detailed conversation with this person about whether you would want to be maintained on a breathing machine and under which circumstances you wouldn't want your life prolonged. Talk about what quality of life means to you. You have to be clear about your goals and values. You can talk about the kind of life you would want to avoid. Do you want life prolonged if you have untreatable pain? What do we do if you suddenly got sick and were on a breathing machine but we didn't think you could get better? But you can also think about quality of life in positive terms, those things that give your life meaning. What in your life is so important to you that you can't imagine living without it?

For some people, a spouse is the likely choice for the role of health care proxy. In fact, if you signed a living will years ago, you may have already assigned this role to your spouse. So you may need to review your will and make sure that this decision still makes sense. A spouse may not be the right choice if he or she cannot make objective decisions for you.

MOLST, POLST Forms

Many patients hire an attorney to create a living will that outlines their goals and values and may even state specific wishes about medical treatment at the end of life. While it's a great idea to do this, you should remember that a living will does not translate into a medical order for treatment. In most states you need to fill out an additional form and have a doctor sign it. This form might be called Medical Orders for Life Sustaining Treatment (MOLST) or Physician Orders for Life Sustaining Treatment (POLST). This form dictates how much treatment you should get in a life-threatening emergency, and that one form is valid no matter where you are—in a hospital or in a rehab facility or at home.

Without one of these forms, you will be considered "full code," meaning that medical professionals must do everything possible to keep you alive, even if you are not conscious and are not likely to regain consciousness. In Massachusetts, the forms are usually bright pink to make them easy for paramedics to find. Once you have filled out a POLST or MOLST form, you should make sure the people who are caring for you can retrieve it easily. Most people don't know that an EMT or emergency room nurse will assume that every patient is full code and attempt resuscitation unless someone can produce these medical orders. People generally keep these forms along with the health care proxy and durable power of attorney in an envelope affixed to the refrigerator and marked as "medical forms." EMTs know to look at the fridge for these forms.

You will want to have a conversation with your oncologist before filling out one of these forms. You can ask directly whether resuscitation (CPR) or intubation will help you as your cancer progresses. Resuscitation is a medical procedure in which the patient receives interventions in the hope of starting the flow of blood and oxygen throughout the body. It involves medication, chest compressions, electric shocks to the chest, and the insertion of a breathing tube. Unfortunately, we know from studies that these medical interventions don't work well in patients who have metastatic cancer (cancer that has spread).

It's unsettling to have to talk about death and to sign a form issuing medical orders. I have to remind patients that signing one of these orders doesn't mean doctors won't do anything for you. Your medical team will still be working to improve your health, to make sure you are as comfortable as possible and free of distress. They can still give you radiation for pain, drain fluid from your lungs, if needed, and give you supplemental oxygen.

Some patients say to me that they want their doctor to make a decision about whether to attempt CPR or insert a breathing tube if they have a medical crisis. Unfortunately, it doesn't work that way. Medical professionals must take life-sustaining measures unless you have filled out this form, even if your quality of life isn't what you want, even if the interventions cause you pain or distress. I caution patients that when you have metastatic cancer, resuscitation probably won't be effective. CPR and intubation won't affect the underlying cancer that has triggered the medical crisis.

Occasionally, a patient will tell me that he or she wants the doctors to try ventilation for a while, and then remove the machines after a few days if things don't get better. It sounds reasonable, and yet most oncologists and palliative care specialists don't recommend short-term ventilation. When you make decisions, you want to think of your family members and what they will be feeling in this situation. Once you are on a ventilator, someone has to decide to remove the machines. And that's a gut-wrenching decision for someone to have to make on your behalf. A growing body of research suggests that when someone's death is prolonged in the intensive care unit, their family members struggle more with grief and with posttraumatic stress.

I suggest that patients ask their doctors several questions. Will the resuscitation allow me to live the quality of life that is acceptable to me? Given what you know about me and about my cancer, what would you recommend? A doctor should give you a recommendation about these kinds of medical interventions just as he or she would recommend medications for you to take.

Implantable Cardiac Defibrillators (ICD)

More and more cancer patients have to consider the issues around a cardiac defibrillator. People who have had heart issues or an irregular heart rhythm may have had a cardiac defibrillator implanted (ICD). This technology can be lifesaving for patients with certain cardiac issues because these defibrillators deliver a shock in the event that the heart goes into a fatal rhythm. For some people the ICD has never needed to deliver a shock to reset the heart's rhythm, while others have experienced several such shocks over the course of many years.

It's easy for patients to assume that the ICD is keeping them alive and that they will die immediately if it is turned off. But this isn't true. The heart will still beat as it does normally without the ICD. It's just that if the heart went into an abnormal rhythm, there would be no shock to correct it.

If you are a patient with advanced cancer who also has an ICD, someone on your medical team may ask whether you want it to be deactivated at some point. The reason they ask is because many patients who are actively dying of cancer will experience a fatal arrhythmia in the final hours of life. This is a very peaceful way to die. If the ICD has not been deactivated, patients will experience a painful shock from the ICD while they are dying. I remember one patient who was in hospice and had an active ICD that shocked him repeatedly in the last two hours of his life. It was actually preventing a natural death for him, something his family found distressing. The family needed to call the hospice nurse to come and deactivate it.

If you have an ICD, you can ask your medical team about the right time to deactivate it. That time could be weeks or months from now, but it is a discussion you want to have.

End of Life Care

I often encourage my patients to start thinking about what they want at the end of life and about the circumstances in which they wouldn't want life prolonged.

There is a growing awareness in our culture that everyone should think and talk about end of life care, what each one of us would want and not want if we had a medical crisis that diminished our quality of life as we see it. But these conversations have even more relevance for patients with advancing cancer.

The Conversation Project is a nonprofit started by journalist Ellen Goodman to help initiate these conversations. The goal of the project is to help people talk about their wishes for end of life care. Goodman started the project after providing end of life care for her mother and realizing that very few people talk to their close family members about what kind of care they would want if their health deteriorated. It starts with asking what your priorities are. Making a statement to your family about what matters to you, what brings you joy in life, is the first step. There are many other questions to answer about how much detail you want about your medical condition and whether you are more afraid of having too much care or too little.

I initiate a lot of these conversations with my patients, and they always help people with cancer to think about what they want and don't want as treatments become more intensive. Sometimes we visit websites together where you can find information about how to determine your goals and values. They think about quality of life and what matters so much to them that they couldn't imagine living without it. There aren't right or wrong answers. Everyone has a different answer to these questions.

My patient Bill told his wife that he wanted to continue to be actively engaged in her life and the lives of their teenaged children. He said that if he was unable to talk or if he had to spend the whole day in bed, he didn't want that type of life prolonged. Whenever he and I discussed potential treatments, he was clear with me that he wanted only those treatments that had a high likelihood of being useful and a low chance of causing symptoms he didn't want, including fatigue, nausea, and pain. He didn't want treatments that would make him too sick to function. He was also clear that he wanted to die at home and that he didn't want any artificial measures to prolong his life. He was able to state what he really wanted, and his wife and I worked to make sure those wishes were carried out.

By contrast, my patient Alexandra, who also had three young children, stated clearly that she wanted every possible medical treatment for her pancreatic cancer, even if that meant suffering on her part. We talked at length about her goals and values. She understood that she would most likely die from her cancer and knew that she didn't want to be resuscitated when she was close to death. Still, she wanted all experimental treatments attempted if they could be safely delivered. Alexandra started a clinical trial a month before her death, even though she had a do not resuscitate order in place and was enrolled in hospice. In the end, Alexandra believed that she had tried every possible medical treatment but also that she had made a plan for the end of her life that would support her and her family.

Choosing Hospice Care

Many people say they hope to die at home if possible, but not everyone wants this. Most patients tell me that they want to be physically comfortable and they don't want to be a burden to their family members. These patients consider the location of death secondary to these other concerns. I think it's great to know what you hope to do, and it's also good to stay flexible if you can't remain at home.

Your care team will encourage you to choose a home hospice provider to give you and your family more support. Hospice gets a bad reputation because so many patients think you can engage hospice only during the final days of life. As a result, they wait too long to get the help that would really be useful. Also, some people think that you have to stop all treatments and stop seeing your regular doctors when you enroll in hospice. This is not true. I like to see my patients every two weeks, even when they are enrolled in hospice, as long as they are feeling strong enough to come to the clinic.

Once you enroll in hospice, that provider pays for all of your medical treatment. This includes medications, nursing and home health aide visits, and any medical equipment such as hospital beds or oxygen. Hospice providers vary in which services they are able to offer. Many smaller hospices can't cover treatments, such as chemotherapy, that can cost $10,000 per month. Larger hospices tend to cover more treatments, and some are considered "open access" providers, meaning that patients can still receive therapies such as chemotherapy and radiation. I know of one hospice in Massachusetts that had more than one hundred patients receiving chemotherapy at one point. Before enrolling in a hospice, do some research to find a provider that can meet your needs. Look for a provider with physicians who are board certified in hospice and palliative medicine.

When to Enroll in Hospice

I often have to explain to patients and families that hospice care is not something just for people who are critically ill or actively dying. It's an insurance benefit available to patients with a likely prognosis of six months or less. (If you live longer than six months, they don't kick you out.) The goal of hospice is to help you live well during these months.

Some patients in hospice have a remarkable amount of energy when they enroll. I had a patient named Kurt with metastatic rectal cancer. He was the kind of guy who loved to split wood and hunt turkeys. He also loved to play the slots at a local casino. His hospice nurse worked with him on taking his medications and managing his energy so that he could get out of the house and spend time with his grandchildren. It's good to think of hospice as a kind of extension of palliative care. Hospice workers want to know your goals and help you live your life. One day, Kurt had so much energy that he went out to play the slots and forgot that his nurse was scheduled to visit him. The nurse was not terribly thrilled about being stood up. In fact, I had to call Kurt about this, and he said, "I know. I'm sorry. But they've got me feeling so good, and I won three hundred bucks."

One reason to enroll in hospice before you think you have a critical need for it is to get to know the people who will be coming to your home. Hospice is a group of providers assigned to you, including doctors, nurses, home health aides, social workers, chaplains, and volunteers. They work best when they have time to learn about your routine so that later on they can provide help more efficiently. A hospice nurse can come to your home up to three times per week, more if necessary, and will spend about an hour each visit. The home health aides can visit you as many as five days a week for about two to three hours at each visit. So, even if you have hospice, you will still rely on family and friends for the majority of your day-to-day needs. Hospice is not twenty-four-hour home care. If you want that kind of care, you have to pay for it out of pocket or consider an inpatient hospice facility.

Inpatient Hospice

Most hospice care happens at home, but you can also receive hospice care in a hospice residence, nursing home, or in the hospital. The care delivered in a hospice residence is similar to the intensity of care that you can receive at home except there are caregivers there all the time to help with cleaning you up, meals, and medications.

Medicare does not cover residential hospice care, so the patient generally has to pay a daily rate. It could be as much as $200 to $500 per day. If you have symptoms that require a lot of monitoring or IV medication, then you need to be in an inpatient hospice facility or in the hospital. Fortunately, these stays are often covered by insurance. Your medical team can help you figure out what kind of care you need.

Some of my patients tour hospice houses to get a sense of where they would feel most comfortable. If you are feeling up to it, this is a great way to help your family decide what kind of care would be best. Your family members may be insisting that you stay at home, and it's wonderful to have a supportive family. Yet, the plan to stay at home doesn't work out for every patient. Sometimes symptoms are too hard to manage for family members. At some point in the future, you may need one or two people with you twenty-four hours a day, and that can be tough for some families to manage. If patients develop delirium or confusion, then caring for them at home can be even more difficult. I like to encourage people to choose a hospice residence or general inpatient hospice unit as a backup plan. You can stay at home knowing that there is another option available if your family members are stretched too thin.

Funerals and Obituaries

Many people say that funerals are for the living, but that doesn't mean you have to leave all the details to others. Some people don't want to think about a possible funeral, but many of my patients have a lot of opinions on the subject. They know whether they want to be buried or cremated. And if they do want to be cremated, they have ideas about where they want their ashes to be scattered. Most people choose a place that has special meaning to them.

If you do have opinions and want them known, you can visit a funeral home to start the planning process. Most funeral homes are very good about helping families manage all these details, including open versus closed casket and planning any wake or memorial service, whether it involves clergy or not. Many of my patients go to the funeral home and pick out the key items such as the casket and help plan the services. If you can pay for the funeral in advance, this will be a great help to family members.

I had a patient with aggressive metastatic breast cancer who was in her early forties. She had lived with her cancer for almost eight years and she really wanted to take charge of her funeral. She also had a quirky sensibility that was reflected in her choices of music, food, and who would speak at the service. She was very close to her niece and encouraged her to perform a funny skit at the funeral. "I want my funeral to be funny and silly like we are as a family," she said to me. "I wrote my obituary, too, and told people that if they can't take a joke, they shouldn't come to the funeral."

Managing Relationships

In the initial chapter on coping (chapter 7), I talked about how to communicate changes in your health status to extended family and friends. It's no different now. You can think of your sphere of relationships as orbits, with an A orbit at the center. Your A orbit is made up of those few people who know your situation well and are the ones providing the most day-to-day support. They know the details of your situation, so you don't have to keep explaining.

The question is how to interact with outer orbits, what I like to call the B or C orbits. These are people you may love a lot and feel close to, but there are only so many times you can tell your story before you start to bore yourself. And, depending on your work history or social history, these outer orbits can consist of a lot of people who check in every few weeks and do want some sort of response or keep asking whether they can help. Be direct about what would be helpful to you and to your family. Maybe you simply want good wishes or prayers. Maybe you need help coordinating transportation or some food. People love to be given specific tasks they can do to help. It allows them to feel involved even when you aren't feeling especially social.

Some of my patients assign someone in the family to serve as an information czar. This is someone who likes writing group e-mails and who is comfortable receiving messages and phone calls from people if they have questions. I usually recommend that this be someone other than a spouse or child of the patient, if possible. Immediate family members need to focus on themselves and the patient, and it can be exhausting to have the same conversation over and over again. If you use a website to manage meal donations or rides, your information czar can be in charge of that as well.

Having Important Conversations

My patients sometimes ask whether they should be thinking about how to communicate love and gratitude to those closest to them. When you have a sense that time might be short, what do you say to the people you love? A few patients want to know whether they should be trying to heal troubled relationships if possible. While there are no right or wrong answers, many palliative care clinicians have written about the kinds of conversations that help people feel some closure about the different relationships in their lives, and this helps them feel less anxious about death. Ira Byock is a palliative care physician who has written several books on this subject, and he believes that these are conversations that everyone should have in order to heal. He identifies five phrases that may be helpful for people to say to loved ones: I'm sorry; I forgive you; thank you; I love you; and good-bye. This can seem formulaic for some people, and this list isn't for everyone. But it does offer a useful guide for how to initiate the kinds of conversations people might be grateful to have.

Legacy Work

Another practical question that patients sometimes ask is about how to create an object or express something to family members that will last. I had a patient who loved doing woodwork. He decided that he wanted to build a cabinet for his wife, a gift of his creativity. Some people want to work on specific projects with children or grand-children, creating photo albums, assembling a family cookbook, or building model cars. Others buy gifts and attach messages to be opened at a significant event, such as a wedding or birthday, or they make videos in which they share memories and messages to loved ones, or they write letters. This is wonderful, meaningful work, but it can also be emotionally difficult, particularly when an illness is advanced and you are struggling with physical symptoms and fatigue. I would never tell anyone that they ought to do this work. It's different for everyone.

People who are very comfortable sharing their thoughts and feelings and have achieved some acceptance that cancer may take their lives at some point may find this work easier. They know that they should do it a little bit at a time on those days when they feel especially strong.

One of my patients decided to write letters to her children in college about six months after her diagnosis. Jane had metastatic lung cancer, and she wanted to start these letters early because she understood how much uncertainty the future held for her, and she wanted to share her thoughts with them and tell them how proud she was of them. Then every six months, she would come into the clinic and say to me, "I wasn't sure I would live this long, but I did. Now I have to rewrite those letters because there is so much more to say." She had a real knack for mock exasperation. We both knew that having to rewrite the letters was a great problem to have.

When writing her letters, Jane focused on highlighting stories about her children and her life that she remembered fondly, and she wrote a lot about what she loved and admired about her children. Although she had ideas about how she wanted them to live, she didn't focus on her own hopes. Children really do want to be seen for who they are and loved for who they are. They can feel burdened by letters filled with expectations about what career path they should choose or what kind of person they should marry. Instead, Jane focused on what it was like to hold each one of them for the first time and what memories of them she cherished most.

22

My Doctor Says That Chemotherapy
Is No Longer Effective

THROUGHOUT THE BOOK, I'VE DESCRIBED how cancer that isn't curable will eventually spread and grow even though you are getting treatment. Every oncologist can tell you that once the cancer has grown through the first and second lines of treatment, the options, unfortunately, become more limited. Even if there are other available drugs, they may work by a mechanism that the tumor has already grown resistant to. Also, the longer you are in treatment, the more likely it is that your body will become weakened from the effects of the cancer and from multiple treatment regimens.

At some point, your oncologist is likely to tell you that continuing with chemotherapy may shorten your life. Or perhaps your doctor will tell you that it simply won't do any good. (This situation is far different from taking a break early on when the treatment is working well. We sometimes refer to those as chemo holidays.)

It's never easy to hear that you won't be getting chemotherapy anymore, but it is possible for chemotherapy to hurt you more than help you. This doesn't mean that you are weak or haven't tried hard enough. It just means that we can't do something that would do more harm than good.

It can be difficult to imagine how chemotherapy could be harmful to you, especially if it has been successful at holding the cancer in check for a long time. Some people demand to continue regimens of chemotherapy even when the doctor has explained that they have a remote chance of lengthening their lives even by a few weeks and when they have a much larger chance of making them sick. People who are dealing with advanced cancer that has caused bone marrow failure and poor kidney or liver function are at higher risk for serious complications from treatment, and this is something oncologists want to avoid.

Even if your oncologist is telling you that you need to stop chemotherapy now, that doesn't mean that you can't have it ever again or that some other disease-modifying treatment won't be helpful to you in the future. In this chapter I'll answer some of the questions that people have at this juncture and give you some guidelines for choosing treatments that are in line with your goals and values.

Are You Giving Up on Me?

Many times this is the first question patients ask their doctors when they are told that chemotherapy is not a treatment option anymore. The answer is absolutely not. Your doctors are still your doctors, and they will still be working with you to manage your cancer and minimize its symptoms.

In some cases, it is even harder for family members to make sense of this new reality. Many oncologists have been confronted by angry family members who say, "I forbid you to tell Dad that there aren't any other treatments." I've been yelled at by spouses, too, who tell me that I've given up on the patient. I feel awful when this happens. I'm not giving up. I just believe that I would be a bad doctor if I didn't prepare my patients and their families for what to expect. I always hope I'm wrong, but I couldn't live with myself if I didn't help people understand what I think could happen if we continue chemotherapy.

How Do You Know Chemotherapy Won't Be Effective?

We have a concept in oncology called performance status (PS). It's a rough rule of thumb that measures how patients feel during treatment. Your doctor will be giving you a PS rating between 0 and 4 at every appointment. If you have no side effects from cancer at all, you have a PS of 0. That means that you wouldn't even know that you had cancer if you weren't in treatment. If you have a PS of 1, you have some symptoms of cancer, but you can still function with good energy, and your daily activities haven't diminished significantly. Once you reach a PS of 2, then you may find that you need to rest off and on during the day, but you are not spending more than half the day resting and conserving energy. A patient who has a PS of 3 is spending more than half the day in bed or on the couch. Once a patient is spending almost the whole day in bed and really struggles to summon the energy to function, that is a PS of 4.

Performance status measures how your body is responding to chemotherapy and how well it is able to bounce back after an infusion. It also serves as a rough measure of tumor burden, meaning the amount of cancer in the body. When patients have a PS of 3 or 4, the tumor burden may be high or the body has been knocked down by chemotherapy. Multiple clinical studies have shown that continuing to give these patients chemotherapy carries enormous risk and that these patients are unlikely to benefit from the treatment. As a result, oncologists are taught from the beginning of training that it's wrong to give chemotherapy to a patient with a PS of 3 or 4 if that patient has a solid tumor.

Hematologic malignancies are different. Patients can often have wonderful responses to chemotherapy even at this performance stage. Therefore, the PS rule usually applies only to patients with solid tumors. We are starting to see a few patients with good responses to targeted therapies and new immunotherapies even with poorer performance status. But these cases are the exception.

What Are My Options?

Sometimes patients know before I do that we've reached this juncture in treatment. They tell me that their fatigue is getting worse again or that they are losing weight. These are the classic signs that cancer is on the move. One of my patients, Dan, had been living with metastatic colon cancer for three years when we got to this point. One day in the clinic he told me that he already knew that the scans were going to show that the cancer was getting worse. He wanted to know what his options were.

This is a good time to have a conversation about treatment options and to ask your oncologist to go over the best- and worst-case scenarios for you. Some people ask, "How long have I got?" But even now an oncologist can't give you a definitive time frame. I told Dan that with colon cancer most people die within six months after chemotherapy stops working but that some people could live for a year or more if their cancer grew slowly.

In terms of other treatments, Dan could try another FDA-approved regimen for colon cancer, but on average it delayed the growth of cancer for only one to two months. He could also do a clinical trial for a drug that worked on his type of cancer in mice, but only ten people had been treated with this drug so far.

I also explained that some people choose to not do any active chemotherapy or clinical trials. Doctors call this supportive care. Many patients worry that this means doctors do nothing, but that's not true. Supportive care means helping patients have a good day each day. That sometimes requires interventions to remove fluid, radiation for pain, or other advanced symptom management. We still have many options to help patients live as well as they can. Your doctor may suggest home hospice at this point, because this will offer your family more support at home and the ability to get medications delivered there.

The next time Dan came in to look at CT scans, he brought his wife, Barbara. She looked grim when he told me that they'd sold their ski condo and he had drawn up a new will. And I knew this discussion was actually for her. For the next hour I explained all the options to Barbara that Dan and I had already discussed. It was a difficult appointment for her, and at first she was insisting that he start the clinical trial right away. Eventually, she agreed that they should go home and discuss it first. We have to remember that there are important goals other than living longer. *How* do you want to live? That is the most critical question at this point.

What Is a Marginally Effective Drug?

When people have exhausted standard chemotherapy, it can be compelling to try some other drug. It can be hard to understand that cancer cells mutate in ways that make them resistant to whole classes of standard treatments. And that means that even promising new drugs may not be effective against cancer cells that have gone through these mutations. Your doctor could try a drug that is FDA approved for another type of cancer, but this is usually not a good idea, because most drugs have already been tested against other types of cancer and have shown little or no benefit. Also, insurance companies often refuse to pay for treatments if the FDA hasn't approved them for your specific type of cancer.

Even if your doctor knows of another line of chemotherapy, he or she may warn you that it will have only a small chance of being effective in your case. Oncologists refer to these drugs as being only marginally effective, meaning that they probably have less than a 10 or 20 percent chance of shrinking the cancer or controlling it for several months. Cancers that have already grown through two or more standard treatments will be far less likely to respond to another line of chemotherapy enough to offer an additional six months of life, and yet this drug will still bring side effects that patients will have to deal with. I always ask patients whether they truly want to do that or whether they want to try a different approach of supportive care.

The thought of stopping treatment may seem unbearable at first, but many people know that they only want to try another regimen with another set of side effects if it's going to be effective in keeping the cancer under control for several months or longer.

What about Experimental Drugs?

Doctors hear this question a lot. When you ask about other drug treatments, your doctor may suggest clinical trials, even phase I trials (see chapter 19), in which drugs are being tested on people for the first time. These drugs will have shown promise in animal models in the lab, and they may be available to you if you qualify for such a study. But the decision to take part in a phase I trial is personal, and you'll want to consider what your goals are beyond the notion of living longer. In many studies of experimental chemotherapy, the goal is to improve longevity, perhaps by a few weeks or months. The goal is not to cure the cancer but to test and measure better treatments.

I had a patient named Mike, who was a seventy-five-year-old engineer with metastatic rectal cancer. He had spent his whole life working for a large engineering firm, and when his tumor had grown through standard chemotherapy options, we had a long talk about whether he should join a phase I study of a novel drug that showed promise in the lab against his type of cancer. The preclinical evidence looked great, but this trial was the first time that people would be taking it. So far, just seven people had tried the drug, and it was too early to see how effective it would be. What impressed me about Mike was that he could look beyond the notion of experimental treatment and think clearly about how he wanted to spend the time he had left. He told me that he had always wanted to build a car with his grandson. He knew that he had four or five good hours each day in which he could focus on a task. Mike told me that if he spent those hours taking a new drug and dealing with the side effects and putting up with the additional testing required by a clinical trial, he wouldn't have enough energy left to build the car. In the end, he said no to the clinical trial, knowing that it was the right decision for him.

What about This Clinic I've Heard about Overseas?

Patients and families sometimes ask whether there are promising drugs in trials overseas, or they ask about experimental treatment regimens in other countries. I had a patient whose son had read about a clinic in Mexico that claimed to be performing miracles with a non-traditional approach to treating cancer. They used a combination of Reiki therapy, massage therapy, nutritional cleanses including coffee enemas, and shark cartilage to treat patients with cancer. It cost $30,000 for a one-week stay. I told the son that I didn't think this was the right thing to do. As a doctor, I am often in a tough spot when patients want to pursue this kind of treatment. There is no data showing that this approach is effective in treating cancer, which is why I recommend against it. I have two major concerns. The first is that traveling to a small clinic in another country could be unsafe and make the patient's life very uncomfortable, and I also deeply worry that the patient could lose his or her life savings on these expensive, unproven treatments. In the end, I can offer only my opinion and my worries. Patients and families make their own decisions.

In this case, the son would not accept my advice, and the patient wanted to keep her family happy, so she agreed to fly to San Diego and then drive down to the clinic. She took out a second mortgage on her condominium in Boston to pay cash for the treatment as the clinic required. When she returned a little over a week later, she was dehydrated and plagued with diarrhea and had lost ten pounds. It took three days to rehydrate her before it was safe to release her from the hospital and into hospice care. Her cancer had not responded at all to these treatments.

Patients can be under enormous pressure from their families to keep fighting using any available experimental treatments. Vicki and I often talk about how to help patients and families see that there is more to this whole cancer experience than just living longer. It is about living *well*. For some patients it is about living longer at all costs, and for those patients no amount of suffering seems like too much. As doctors, this is difficult to watch. It just feels wrong to cause harm, and we don't feel comfortable prescribing treatments that will make people worse.

But I Can Still Beat This, Right?

When people are pushing hard to do more chemotherapy or try experimental treatments, there is often something at work behind this demand. Vicki and I sometimes refer to this as the tyranny of positive thinking. Some people tell themselves that if they can believe in and visualize a different future for themselves, they can change their own biology. Some people tell themselves that they can stop their cancer cells from growing if they have the right attitude. When patients or family members say this to me, I get worried.

I would never discount the power of positive thinking. Cancer patients and their families go through so much in treatment, and many of them do it with such grace and strength—even humor—that Vicki and I feel lucky to know them. We know they aren't battling the cancer itself but rather fighting to have as much of a normal life as they can despite this terribly unfair diagnosis and despite difficult treatment regimens. They have needed to stay positive and to believe in themselves to do all of that, and it's hard to express how much I admire this fortitude.

And yet I worry about people who tell me that they know they will be cured if they just keep believing that this is true. I've had crying patients tell me that their cancer has grown because they didn't stay positive enough, and that breaks my heart because it's not true. You can't wish cancer away. I've often been stopped outside an exam room or hospital room by a family member who forbids me to tell the patient that the cancer is getting worse. "You aren't going to tell Mom that this is incurable, are you? You aren't going to tell her that she might die?" I've been asked some version of these questions many times. Some family members tell me that the patient has to believe that he or she will be cured in order to be cured.

Hope is an essential part of being human, and I would never tell anyone to give up hope. I hope, too, that every patient will be the exception. I just want patients and family members to hold onto hope while still being able to understand the medical facts and to understand something about how the disease is likely to progress. This gives patients the chance to focus on the task of finding ways to live well.

By having this understanding, patients and family members can also make better decisions about what kind of treatments they want and don't want. For example, if a bone marrow transplant brings a 70 percent chance of cure for a patient's leukemia, that patient may choose to undergo this arduous procedure knowing that it has a real likelihood of allowing a good quality of life for years or decades afterward. When we say that a certain drug has a less than 10 percent chance of shrinking a tumor that we know won't ever be cured, or if it will likely extend life by only a couple of weeks, the patient might reasonably choose not to try it. I need to give my patients a realistic framework for understanding their illness and their treatment options. This is the heart of informed consent.

Living Two Weeks Longer Is Better, Isn't It?

Some people wonder whether extending life by any length of time is an appropriate goal for them. This is a great question to consider when deciding on an experimental treatment. Researchers are always testing new drugs to see whether they extend longevity and by how much.

One recent example was with the drug erlotinib, which inhibits the epidermal growth factor pathway. Some tumors exploit this pathway in order to keep growing. When used against lung cancers that harbor a mutation of the epidermal growth factor receptor, erlotinib is astonishingly effective. A patient at Mass General has been on erlotinib for more than ten years even though he has metastatic lung cancer. His tumor shrank and can't grow back as long as he's taking it. He is an exceptional case. Most people get a year or two of great quality of life before the drug stops working. Researchers were so excited about this response that several studies tested it against other cancers, such as pancreatic cancer.

The National Cancer Institute of Canada performed a large phase III clinical trial in which half of pancreatic cancer patients received standard chemotherapy and the other half received that same standard chemotherapy plus erlotinib. The study results showed that patients who received the erlotinib lived on average two weeks longer than patients who received standard chemotherapy alone. The results were statistically significant, but this doesn't mean that this drug is going to make a meaningful difference in any one patient's life.

Is adding an average of two weeks of life significant for any individual patient? It would be if the drug were free of side effects.

Erlotinib often triggers a severe rash on the face, diarrhea, and can occasionally cause shortness of breath. That's why most people don't take erlotinib unless they have lung cancer with that specific gene mutation.

What Would You Advise Your Mother or Father to Do in This Situation?

Oncologists hear this question a lot from patients. Some of them hate to have to answer it, but I love this question. I know it's incredibly valuable to my patients as they navigate the difficult choices they have to make. It's no different from asking a lawyer or an accountant or any other expert what he or she would do in your situation. I generally frame my answers by describing my parents. My mother is a devoutly religious woman who raised seven children. She hates the idea of chemotherapy and would never agree to it just to live a couple of extra months. She has said to me that if the good Lord wants her to live longer, he is in charge of that. My father, on the contrary, was a bit of a risk taker. He might have taken a chance on a new experimental clinical trial that offered the possibility of a sustained response. What I hope to explain to patients by talking about my parents is that there are no correct answers, only correct answers for you. The best way to make the right decision is to know what kind of person you are and how you want to live.

For every patient with advanced, incurable cancer, there will come a point when taking a break from chemotherapy is the right thing to do. Supportive care and helping patients to feel as well as they can become the focus of good care. It may be easier to focus on chemotherapy rather than on the business of living. It's certainly easier for the oncologist, who can talk about abstract issues such as response rates and overall survival. I want patients to focus more on what they want to do with the time they have left.

23

My Body Feels Like It's
Shutting Down

AS PEOPLE START TO FEEL more fatigued and spend more time in bed
during the day, they wonder what the process of dying from cancer
is like. How is it going to feel? Am I going to know when it's happening? Does it take a long time?

This is not an easy subject to think about or read about. People
who aren't dealing with cancer often want to avoid thinking or talking about death, but so often patients do want to know how they will
be taken care of and kept comfortable during the time when they are
actively dying. Some people take great comfort in knowing what
might happen next and how diligently the hospice team, the oncology team, and the palliative care team will be working to help them
at this time.

In this chapter, I'll describe the possible outcomes as cancer continues to progress. The first thing to know is that for most people
with cancer, dying can be peaceful. Most people decline gradually
and die in their sleep, and this is true even if they die of liver failure
or infection. As people get closer to death, the hospice team can help
patients and their families know what to expect and explain the
many ways to help minimize discomfort or distress, even in the final

hours of life. Of course, there are some instances where patients have an acute change in status, where they go from feeling relatively stable to needing hospitalization or admission to an inpatient hospice facility to get the kind of medical care that wouldn't be possible at home. If you are hoping to stay home during this time, you'll need a lot of support from family and friends, and I'll describe why. At the same time, you may be wondering how to manage information that goes out to extended family and friends or how many people you want visiting you at this time. We can talk about ways that other people have handled these issues.

But I also remind patients that they aren't dying yet. I've worked with people who have been in hospice care for a couple of months who say to me, "I can't believe that I'm still here." It can be tricky to figure out how to keep setting goals and keep finding things to look forward to, but you can do this.

For many people, spiritual issues become more pronounced even for those who are not sure they believe in God or an afterlife. Hospitals have chaplains or a chaplaincy service that can help people talk through any spiritual questions that they may have.

How Will I Die?

Throughout this book, I've said that your medical team members may not be able to give you an exact time frame for how long you will live. But your oncologist should be able to tell you whether you are in the last six months of life. For most types of cancer, doctors know on average how long people live after each stage of treatment. This is a good time to ask your oncologist to give an approximate time frame for death. I tell patients to do this because having some idea of whether you might live a few weeks, a few months, or more than six months can help you think about how you want to live during that time.

You can also ask your oncologist how you might die. A few oncologists may not like to hear these questions and may dismiss them because this is hard to talk about. Many oncologists welcome these questions and any chance to talk to you about your wishes during the dying process. I've found that people are sometimes worried about asking these questions and hearing the answers but then find the conversation actually eases their fears and helps them to make relevant decisions and have important conversations with their loved ones.

Typically, death comes by one of several pathways. It is either a slow decline caused by the cancer or a more sudden acute process caused either by the cancer or by treatment.

The Slow Decline

The most common way that people die from cancer is in a decline that occurs over many months. The patient becomes gradually more fatigued and spends more of the day in bed or asleep and begins to lose interest in eating. Although there may be pain or nausea or other symptoms, these are dependent on the location of any tumors and aren't universal.

The goal of the medical team is still to help you have a good quality of life, which means to be alert and comfortable. Sometimes your doctor may want to give medications to control symptoms even though they cause sedation. If the symptoms are difficult to control, you may need to trade comfort for alertness, but I always ask patients what they want. Do they want to be more alert to interact with family, or do they really want the pain to be minimized? Continuing to communicate your goals is paramount.

I treated April, who was a seventy-two-year-old woman with breast cancer. She had a terrific response with hormonal therapy for the first four years of treatment. Over the next couple of years, when the first therapy stopped working, she tried other antiestrogen therapies that were less successful. In her seventh year of treatment, she knew that her pain and fatigue were getting worse and that she was losing weight, no matter what she ate. Her doctor tried several rounds of chemotherapy, but they didn't control the tumors. Eventually, she lost her appetite as well and knew that she was near the end of effective treatment.

April didn't want to disappoint her oncologist, who had been treating her from the beginning, so she asked her palliative care specialist what dying would be like and when it might occur. She was an immensely practical person who had lost her husband several years earlier, and so she knew what she needed to do to get her estate in order and signed an advance health directive and even made plans to travel while she could. Then she told her oncologist that she was done with chemotherapy and not interested in a clinical trial. She wanted to be enrolled in hospice, where she became quite friendly with her hospice nurse. For the next couple of months, she still came in to see the oncologist every two weeks and had her medications adjusted when she had new symptoms. She told her medical team that she was at peace with what was happening. Gradually, she became more fatigued and had to miss an appointment. After that, it became clear that she needed help around the clock, because she had trouble getting to the bathroom on her own. Her children began taking turns sleeping at her house. Soon, she informed them that she wanted inpatient hospice care, which her nurse helped arrange for her. The next day an ambulance picked her up, and she moved with two suitcases to the hospice facility. She was soon bedbound and told me that she couldn't believe how fatigued she was. The hospice facility managed her pain and kept her comfortable, and in the third week she drifted into a coma and died forty-eight hours later with her family present.

During a slow decline, patients have time to take care of practical and personal matters. They see the cancer getting worse in multiple ways and gradually accept the prognosis (the likely course and outcome of their disease) and the inevitability of death. April was lucky to have both an oncologist and a palliative care physician with whom she could speak about her wishes. And she was lucky to have a supportive family, people who were available to stay with her when she needed help. April was also lucky in that she had a great awareness of her prognosis. Each step along the way she understood what the goals of treatment were and how they interacted with her overall goals of care. So she was able to choose an inpatient hospice facility when she didn't want her family members to feel that they had to bear sole responsibility for caring for her.

While we hope that every patient has such a comfortable and gentle death, complications from cancer and treatment can occur at any step and turn a chronic process into an acute or subacute process. That's why it is so important to acknowledge the possibility of death if you can shortly after diagnosis. People are sometimes afraid to think about this subject because they don't want other people to think that they are giving up. Sometimes they don't want the oncologist to think that they're giving up. Acknowledging the possibility of death is not equivalent to giving up. In all my years of caring for patients who are dying from cancer, I've rarely had anyone who didn't want more time.

Subacute Decline

This is a medical event that can occur when patients have already begun to experience fatigue and other symptoms of advancing cancer. Patients can go from feeling relatively stable to being close to death over the course of a few weeks or days. It's less common than the slow decline, but patients should be aware that it can happen. Cancers of the pancreas and lung and melanoma are notorious for speeding their growth suddenly, even after many months of being held in check. A few small metastatic nodules can become large metastases in the liver or lungs in just a few weeks. Hematologic cancers can also rapidly worsen seemingly all of a sudden.

For years, a colleague of mine treated Nancy for a slow-growing chronic lymphocytic leukemia that came under control every time she tried chemotherapy. Every time she noticed more fatigue or swelling in the lymph nodes of her neck, she would come in to see her oncologist, who would treat her with chemotherapy. Almost within a week of starting therapy, she would feel better and her symptoms would disappear. Her treatment went on like this for eight years, until one day the symptoms didn't go away. Her oncologist took some scans and found that her indolent cancer had spread quickly to her liver, lungs, and abdomen. Her oncologist suspected that her leukemia had become an aggressive lymphoma, and a biopsy confirmed this.

Nancy decided to try a more aggressive chemotherapy regimen, and she told her oncologist that she had a lot of living to do but wasn't sure it was in the cards. She tolerated the chemotherapy well but after a few rounds was admitted to the hospital with a fever and extreme fatigue. She told her doctor right away that the chemotherapy wasn't working. He took some more scans and confirmed that her liver and kidneys were on the verge of shutting down. Her doctor stabilized her and made her comfortable and then sent her home with hospice care and the support of her family. Nancy died within ten days of leaving the hospital.

Nancy was fortunate that she had several years of slow-growing cancer, and she and her family knew that at some point the cancer would not be controlled by treatment anymore. Still, the sudden change in her condition was something they struggled to cope with.

Many times, people have been in treatment for far less time before the cancer begins this faster growth, and this dramatic change in circumstances can be difficult to understand. In these cases of subacute decline, it is important to keep communicating with your medical team about what is happening, what treatment options are available, and how your plan for dying at home may need to give way to a plan B in which you get medical support during the final days if necessary.

Even if your doctor told you that you could hope for an additional six to twelve months of a gradual decline, that may not be possible if the cancer begins to move more aggressively or if a truly acute event happens. In these cases, communication among family members is crucial. Without it, some family members can panic and begin to argue over the next steps in treatment for the patient. There is always uncertainty in cancer treatment, which is why in palliative care we work with people to have important conversations about end of life care, because they can become relevant without warning.

The Acute Decline

Occasionally, a patient with cancer can develop a life-threatening condition within a few hours and without much warning. Thankfully, this is uncommon. These acute problems stem either from the cancer or from the treatment and can trigger a hospitalization and initiate the process of dying.

Most of the time, acute events result from bleeding or clotting issues. A patient can have a blood clot go to the lungs or brain, or a major blood vessel can start to bleed. While these events can occur at any time during cancer treatment, they are more likely to happen after the treatments have stopped working.

Dave had a patient named Don who had lived with metastatic colon cancer for four years and had been through several lines of chemotherapy. Don knew that his cancer was progressing, and he had already talked about the possibility of enrolling in home hospice or starting a clinical trial. Don had asked about his best-case scenario, and Dave had told him that he was likely to die in the next few months.

One day, Don experienced sudden, severe chest pain and difficulty breathing. Don's wife brought him to the emergency room, and doctors found that a massive blood clot had traveled from his pelvis to his lungs before dividing into multiple smaller clots. It was clear that his lungs and heart were already starting to shut down. Dave had tried before to talk to him and to his wife about his wishes for end of life care, but they had put these discussions off. Now, Don told Dave that he didn't want to die in the intensive care unit. He knew that even if he had a breathing tube inserted, he was unlikely to ever leave the hospital and would probably never come off the ventilator. Don decided that he wanted comfort management alone, which meant that he would receive morphine and other medications to ease the work of breathing. He was admitted to a private room in the hospital where his family could be alone with him. Soon, he drifted off to sleep but could still be aroused by questions from his wife and children. He could nod or shake his head to questions and smile at his family. Over the next few hours, his breathing pattern changed and became irregular. Doctors call this Cheyne-Stokes, which is a breathing pattern of slow, deep breaths followed by shallow, quick breaths. It's common as patients approach death but doesn't signal any distress or pain. Don looked peaceful, and nurses continued to check on him to adjust his medications. Don died comfortably later that evening surrounded by his wife and children.

When an acute event happens early in treatment, such as bleeding in the gastrointestinal system or in the lungs, doctors will do everything possible to stop the bleeding and get people back into treatment. But when these events occur after someone has exhausted several rounds of chemotherapy, we usually have conversations about how to treat them if they happen again. There is usually an option to try to stop the bleeding, but sometimes people tell their doctors that they want to be made comfortable if something irreversible happens. In that case, the patient can be admitted to the hospital, where the medical team will have the goal of minimizing discomfort.

People who have brain metastases can have acute neurologic events, in which a stroke or a new lesion (tumor) can render them confused and disoriented. Brain metastases (tumors spread to the brain) can sometimes cause seizures. If this happens, doctors usually admit the patient to the hospital because it is difficult for families to manage these situations at home. Even if this happens, the medical team will work to keep the patient comfortable and help family members understand what's happening.

Help at Home

At this point in treatment, when fatigue becomes much more pronounced, doctors recommend home hospice care, which is a medical benefit that allows you to get extra care in your home. Most insurance policies cover this care. To qualify for home hospice, two doctors have to certify that they believe you have a prognosis of less than six months. Even if the doctors are wrong and you live longer than six months, you won't be kicked out. Many people think that hospice care is for people who are actively dying, but that's not true. This crucial benefit can help you when you may have months to live.

Hospice does not provide twenty-four-hour care in the home; rather, it allows for home visits from a nurse, and it allows you to get medications delivered to your home. You are required to have a weekly visit from a nurse, but you can have visits more often if needed, and most hospice providers offer a team, including social workers, who can offer emotional support to you and your family. There are chaplains who can visit you at home if you don't feel well enough to attend services. Home health aides can come to your house three to five days a week for a couple of hours at a time to help with daily living tasks. Many hospice services also engage volunteers who can come to your home and spend time with you while a loved one runs an errand.

I usually suggest that people start with some home health aide help. This allows you to get used to someone coming to your house while you can still care for yourself. You can teach the home health aide how to best assist you, and you can figure out whether the home health aide is a good fit for you. Also, most people don't know how much their loved ones worry about leaving them alone. Family members sometimes don't confess their fears to the patient and end up feeling trapped in the house. Having a home health aide stop by for an hour or two can free them to do errands and take a break.

Even if you have engaged home hospice, you might need more support than you think you do. I often suggest making a plan to have friends and family in the home around the clock. If you've lived alone, this might be a good time to have family members stay in the house or to stay at a friend or family member's home. Your health status can change abruptly, but it will also change gradually, and you don't know when you might begin to have more trouble getting to the bathroom, staying hydrated, or even getting in and out of bed.

Eating and Drinking

At this point, many patients don't have much interest in eating. Doctors don't worry about whether the patient is eating food, but many family members want the patient to continue to eat, even if he or she can get only a few bites down at a time. It can become a real battle as loved ones insist that eating is important to keep up strength. I tell patients that you don't have to eat or drink to please anyone and it's not going to keep up your strength. In some cases, trying to eat when you don't feel like it can actually make you feel sick. Your body is giving you signals that it doesn't need much food or that it can't process food in the way it did before.

Doctors also don't recommend appetite stimulants at this point, such as megestrol acetate (Megace) or dronabinol (Marinol). And there is usually no reason to give extra fluids through an IV. When your body is slowing down, IV fluids can make you feel miserable, and sometimes the fluid pools in the stomach or lungs in a way that would require a procedure to drain it. This is the time to listen to your body's natural signals.

You Aren't Dying Yet

I often have to remind patients that they are still living with cancer. My role in palliative care is to help people live as well as they can, even when their bodies are slowing down and cancer treatments have stopped. There will come a time when you are in the last days or hours of life, but that hasn't happened yet. You still want to work to make sure that your symptoms are well treated. You may feel limited in your choice of activities, but you are still living and setting goals about how you want to spend your final weeks in ways that allow you to grow and think and connect with others.

My patient Bonnie was a master at this. She found a variety of things she could do depending on her energy level. Some days she listed to podcasts of interesting topics or stories, such as *The Moth Radio Hour* or *This American Life*. Some days she felt up to reading. She and her daughters had read novels together throughout her illness. Their book group gave them something to talk about other than the illness and the uncertain future. This last phase of her life was no different. On days when she felt really crummy, she had videos cued up to watch that made her laugh or about topics that were interesting to her. Her friends and family kept her engaged and learning even in this final phase of her life. Another patient, Jenny, binged on every season of *Breaking Bad* in the last eight weeks of her life. She was hooked on that show, and it gave her something to distract herself and also to chatter with others about.

My patient George had been living for a long time with pancreatic cancer when he got to this point. At sixty-two, he had an extended family with grown kids and growing grandchildren. He knew that he wanted to be with his family as much as possible and to be somewhere outside. He wanted to be able to return work e-mails when he felt good enough. At the same time, he had physical symptoms that needed medical attention. He had fluid building in his abdomen that needed to be drained every day. So we helped him engage with a hospice facility on the shore where he and his wife owned a small cottage, and he stayed in that cottage, near the beach that he loved. There he held court with family and friends. He had a great time, resting when he needed to, eating a little bit when he felt able. On some days he was awake more, and on some days he slept or rested for much of the day. When a couple of his kids participated in an annual race to benefit a local cancer charity, George attended the race in his wheelchair and cheered them on.

We also had a medical plan in place in case he needed acute medical care, even if he didn't want to die in the hospital. He knew that he could be admitted to a hospital with an inpatient hospice facility. George found a way to stay connected and to make choices that were meaningful to him about how to spend this time. That's what I say to my patients. This phase is sort of a marathon, not a sprint. We don't know how this is going to play out, and there are still going to be good days for you.

For many people, spending time with friends and family feels critically important, and yet they worry about people sitting in some sort of vigil. They ask me whether it's okay to laugh and whether it's okay just to be together without talking much. Of course it is. You can still forget about the illness and concentrate on spending time together.

One of my patients asked his grown children to lug all the photo boxes out of the attic, so that they could go through them together. Gene had just a couple of hours each day when he felt energetic, but they would spend that time looking at photos and retell the old stories behind them. On the days that he didn't feel up to this, he would watch classic baseball games, especially his recording of the Red Sox winning the World Series.

The key is to find the balance between pushing yourself to engage in the world and resting when you need to. On days when you feel like you can swing it, get up and come into the world. Make plans for how you are going to spend the day. Maybe it is reading or visiting with a friend. These goals are probably quite different from the goals that you had when you were well, but it is vital to have them.

Communicating with Others

Some people wonder about how to communicate with extended family and friends about their illness. We've talked about how to do that at the time of diagnosis, but some people are uncertain about how to communicate changes in their health status or how to let people know that visitors are more or less welcome at this time.

I always remind people to think of friends and family in terms of orbits. Your A orbit consists of those people who are closest to you, the people who have offered the most help and support at home and those who bring energy and joy into your life. These folks probably already know most of the details of your situation.

People in outer orbits, we might call them B or C orbits, know far less about your prognosis. Some may know very little about it. They love you, and many of them want to know more about how to help and how to offer support to your family. They might even want to send notes or call, but they don't know what's okay and what would be intrusive. It can be helpful to find a way to communicate some details about how you are doing and offer some guidelines about how these people can help or communicate with you if they want.

Some people choose to write a group e-mail or post on a Caring Pages blog that they can update as circumstances change. Someone in your A orbit can help you do this or can be assigned to send out an e-mail that you write. Be sure to think about how you want people to be in touch with you if they want to, and state whether you want to have visitors and when those visits would be welcome. Seeing old friends and extended family can sometimes feed your energy level, but it can also deplete your energy. Or, as one patient put it to me, "So many people want to come and see me before I die. It's nice." And then she added drily, "My nephew's fiancée, though—I could have done without that one." Even if you aren't up to a lot of visitors, people might be encouraged to send notes or e-mails sharing their memories and good wishes that you can read on your own time.

I've attached a letter that a patient of mine wrote to his family. I love this letter because Alexander is so open about what's happening and yet he is clear about the love and gratitude that he has for his life and for the people who will be reading the letter. You don't have to write a letter like this, but it can be useful to see how others have handled this type of communication. Alexander and his family gave me permission to share this letter. He told me that after he sent it, he received the most powerful response from his extended network of friends. People were deeply touched by the letter, and many wrote to him to say so.

Dear Friends,

I sit here at dusk, looking out of a genuinely lovely room at MGH, and think of how deeply fortunate I am to have you all, my wife Lisa, my boys, my home, the beauty of this sunset over the Charles, and the many relationships and experiences that have made my life as rich and wonderful as it is. I am happy with my life and have lived well, without regret.

As many of you know, my year-and-a-half battle with this uncommon gastrointestinal cancer has had its ups and downs, during which I have received extraordinary care from MGH and, as needed, Dana-Farber Cancer Institute. Through October I had been coping with the gradual spread of the cancer reasonably enough. However, last Wednesday I had a PET scan (nuclear medicine that highlights locations of likely cancerous activity) and a CT scan (more detailed imaging of bone, muscle, and tissue) that displayed a thoroughly new picture of my body. Unfortunately, Wednesday's scans showed an aggressive spread into my hips, back, pelvis, lungs, and brain, with several ribs fractured due to the disease and a blood clot in a lung, which whisked me back into the hospital for immediate attention and monitoring.

And so I have turned the corner into my last chapter. We have known this was coming—my cancer was identified some time ago as uncurable—but we did not expect as sudden a shift as this. So we will accommodate it, as we have each setback along the way that this cancer has presented. The surprise was for my boys, William, sixteen, and Andrew, thirteen. We told them on Saturday afternoon in perhaps the toughest moment our family has ever had. They have always known the uncurable aspect of my cancer and were aware all treatments had failed, but we had not previously introduced the soon-to-be-fatal feature of my cancer—out of respect to let them live their teenage lives without the cloud of my imminent death constantly over their heads. They also were not fully aware my demise would be so soon: months, not years. I now have probably two to six weeks to live; my doctors still find it difficult to identify and forecast how the spreading cancer will bring my days to an end.

My boys are strong and courageous, and Lisa is a rock. Our afternoon meeting was traumatic, and it was but the start of a long process to absorb loss and grief and again move forward. I have full faith that the three of them will find a path back to happiness, however they construct that, and find a way to celebrate my memory, feel my ongoing love, and know that their lives hold plenty of joy, challenge, beauty, and satisfaction across the years ahead.

I expect to be discharged from MGH today, after some further radiation to kill pockets of cancer in my hips and back, where it could still do painful damage in a short time. I will also return for specialized radiation that aims to kill the two small tumors in my brain, which could also cause trouble if untreated. My discharge will be to hospice care at home, which has long been our plan, and I will stay at home so long as it works well for all. If I need to be in a facility, I will enter a lovely one in Danvers, Massachusetts, that is the inpatient location for the at-home hospice organization Care Dimensions.

My energy is low, and some days I get only three to four really good hours in the morning and then a drowsy afternoon and evening focused on pain management, as the evenings and overnights are usually my most challenging. I would love to see so many of you as your own schedules permit, and maybe that will work for us in many instances. But I do tire easily, and I have yet to see what my decline over this period at home or in Danvers will be like, so I'm keeping my expectations modest. I always value and appreciate an e-mail, a card, or a poem; and phone calls are good but too can be tiring, depending on how the day is going.

I am so grateful for the support, care, and love you have shown me. I am sorry my life has to end now and curtail the relationships that have made, and continue to make, my existence the rich, fun, exciting, and worthy journey it's been. There are silver linings everywhere, if you know to look for them, and I have grown immensely in the past nineteen months. I wouldn't wish this experience, or this premature death, on anybody, but some of the new closeness, deepened relationships, revelations of character, and demonstrations of love I have received have left me moist-eyed at what my friends have done for me and what good people will do for each other.

Thank you. It is a genuine pleasure to have spent the time we have. Stay well. Please reach out to my wife and boys over the months and years after I'm gone. And when you do, remember me with a smile.

Yours,

Alexander

24

What Is a Good Death?

MANY PEOPLE TELL ME THAT they want a good death. For most people that means they hope to be free of pain or other discomfort and to be surrounded by the people they love. They also hope to have achieved some acceptance about their own death. Everyone has a different idea of what a good death would be. Some people do want to be at home during their final days and hours, and others feel that having daily physical care being done by family is unthinkable because they don't want their immediate family to feel burdened or stressed.

As difficult as it might be to think about and talk about death, Vicki and I find that articulating what they want at the end of life helps many patients feel more in control. Also, how someone dies is part of how they lived. The person who is dying should have some say in what happens and where it happens. It's also important for families to hear the patient's wishes. Not every wish of a dying patient can be carried out. Sometimes your medical condition can get complicated, and you will need more care than you can get at home or at a residential facility to stay comfortable while you are actively dying. In this chapter, I'll outline some of the issues that people should think about when having these conversations about how to have a good death.

Dying at Home

I worked with a patient early in my career who had metastatic breast cancer that had spread to her liver. Monica was seventy-nine and had an extended family that included her husband, five children, and seventeen grandchildren. She also had several siblings with large families. Her grandchildren were old enough to take turns sleeping in a cot next to Monica's bed so they could help her get to the bathroom in the middle of the night. Her last days were spent playing cards or having people read to her. In the rest of the house, people gathered after work or school to share stories. Walking into that house always made me happy, because it was filled with love and kindness. I remember saying to Monica that I hoped my death would be like this, in a home filled with people laughing and talking. Monica had minimal pain and greeted everyone with a smile. Gradually she lost energy and drifted into a coma that lasted for about twelve hours before she died peacefully in her sleep.

Monica was lucky in several ways. First, her symptoms were easy to control. She didn't suffer from delirium or confusion, and she didn't have a lot of pain or dizziness or shortness of breath. Second, she had an extended family of healthy adults who wanted to care for her. Her grandchildren had extra time and energy to help by spending the night with her and taking care of her daily tasks, including helping her to the bathroom, helping her wash herself, changing her sheets, and getting whatever bites of food she felt able to eat. Third, the patient and her family understood that she was dying and that the purpose of treatment was to keep her comfortable. If you took away one or two of these factors, dying at home would not have been possible for Monica or any other patient.

I know that, in palliative care, clinicians ask specific questions of patients who say they want to die at home. No one wants a patient to go home to a situation that's untenable for the family or one that isn't safe. If you are in a hospital and want to be discharged to your home to die, your medical team will want to talk about several factors.

Have you enrolled in hospice care? It is essential to have medical professionals involved who are experts in end of life care. In addition, you may need to hire additional home health aides, and if so, you'll want to know what the cost would be.

Are your symptoms well controlled? Your doctor will want to be re-assured that your pain is under control with medication, that you can come in if you need fluids drained from your lungs, and that you are medically stable enough to leave the hospital. No one wants your family to suffer through a medical crisis at home in which your symptoms flare and you become distressed. The goal is to make sure you can die at home while staying peaceful and comfortable.

How much help is available at home? You need adults staying with you in the house who can help with washing, toileting, and preparing any food. Hospices require that patients have someone with them at all times. What most people don't realize about hospice is that it is not twenty-four-hour care. The lion's share of the care falls to family caregivers. Providing this kind of care for a loved one is hard, and it works best if there are several people to take turns staying with you, and you might need two people inside the house at all times. That sounds like a lot of help, and it is, but it's a good benchmark to make sure that there are enough adults around who can give breaks to immediate family members. Otherwise, it is just too hard to provide the appropriate care. This is why dying at home doesn't work for everyone.

Are there any other issues that would make home care difficult? If a patient is struggling with confusion or delirium or if he or she is not able to stand because of dizziness or unable to cross the room even with assistance because of shortness of breath, a doctor might wonder whether dying at home is still possible. I know of one palliative care clinician who cared for her mother-in-law at home while she was in the advanced stages of pancreatic cancer. Although the mother-in-law was an independent woman who was able to care for herself throughout her illness, in the end she struggled with dizziness from her medications. This became worse as her liver function declined and her body wasn't able to metabolize medication easily. She fell several times and then developed confusion. My colleague is a medical professional in palliative care who truly wanted to help her loved one and care for her in a home setting, but in this case the best option for the patient was a residential treatment facility where she could get the care she needed.

Dying at a Residential Hospice

Sometimes the family isn't nearby, or the patient doesn't feel comfortable having loved ones taking on the burden of care. Sometimes the illness doesn't allow for patients to die at home.

If dying at home isn't possible, some people choose a residential hospice. Think of this as a setting that feels more like home than a hospital. In a residential hospice, nurses and aides can care for you twenty-four hours a day. It's not the same intensity of care as you will find in a hospital, but there are nurses and aides available all the time.

Tim was a thirty-eight-year-old patient that Vicki treated. He had lived with a slowly progressing brain tumor for nine years, and, in the last three months of his life, he needed a great deal of physical care. He had severe headaches and daily seizures. Tim's wife, Colleen, had two children to care for at home, and she worked full time. She knew that she couldn't be Tim's primary caretaker in the final phase of his illness. The rest of Tim's family lived on the other side of the country and couldn't leave everything to offer months of help. So Tim moved into a residential hospice for two months at the end of his life. In most cases, families need to pay a daily rate at such a facility. It is usually a sliding scale between $200 and $500 a day. Vicki helped Colleen to petition his health insurer to pay his daily fee, because the residential hospice offered better and less expensive care than he would receive in a nursing home.

Colleen told Vicki that she felt incredibly supported by the residential hospice. It was nearby, so she could stop there on the way to work and on the way home. She brought the kids in, and they spent all day Saturday and Sunday with Tim. They came to know the staff well. In the final days of Tim's life, Colleen took time off from work and spent whole days with him, and yet she was able to be there as his wife and not as his primary caregiver, which was important to her. She said she knew that if the kids needed her, she could take care of them knowing that the nurses and aides who knew Tim would be taking care of him. He died peacefully surrounded by his family and by the staff who had become like family.

Dying in an Inpatient Hospice

For some patients, dying in a hospital setting might be the best choice. When patients have symptoms that are difficult to control, such as nausea, confusion, or pain, the intensive treatment available at the hospital may be the best approach to keep them comfortable and free of distress.

Vicki had a patient named Don who lived with a rare and aggressive form of lung cancer. Don was fifty-four and had never married or had children. His elderly parents, who lived six hours away from him, were his closest relatives, and he had chosen his best friend to be the agent of his health care proxy. He might have been a good candidate for a residential hospice, except that his pain was difficult to treat in the last phase of his illness. He needed IV pain medication, and the doses had to be frequently adjusted to keep him comfortable.

In the last weeks of his life, Don moved into a nice inpatient hospice facility paid for by his insurance. There he basically held court for a large retinue of friends. On nice days, the staff wheeled him out to the garden so he could chat or watch the birds. And he felt confident that the staff could manage his pain. Don stopped talking about four days before his death. He slept deeply and roused occasionally to signal the staff if he felt pain. He died peacefully in his sleep surrounded by his friends and his elderly parents.

Dying in the ICU

Vicki and I spend a lot of time talking to patients who have advanced cancer about preparing for the possibility of death and taking care of practical matters and thinking about where they would like to be when they die. We do this because we hope patients can form a plan for what to do if the cancer gets worse. We also do it because we want patients to avoid dying in the intensive care unit if possible. All cancer specialists and palliative care specialists have worked with patients who refuse to think about death and refuse to make any plan for it. And by the time the cancer progresses to the point that it is affecting multiple systems in their bodies—their liver and kidney function, their bowels, their lungs—they don't have options for the kind of medical care that would allow them to die peacefully with family and friends nearby. When a medical crisis arises, they have to go to the hospital ICU, where they receive intensive treatments that are uncomfortable, even painful, and distressing for their families. And none of these intensive end of life treatments do anything to modify the cancer that caused the crisis. Death in the ICU is often traumatic for all involved. Doctors recommend medical interventions that have a good chance of helping the patient to feel better and to live longer, if possible. These include medications to minimize discomfort or treat infection. Unfortunately, if someone is dying from cancer, putting that person on a breathing machine or performing CPR (resuscitation) will not improve quality of life. In fact, it may extend life for only a short time.

Doctors know that people want to live as fully as they can for as long as they can. But, when they are dying, they don't want that process to be prolonged or uncomfortable. So, when doctors see patients with metastatic cancer die in the ICU, we consider it a bad death because we know it could have been more peaceful.

Will My Family Be Okay during This Last Phase?

Family members will need extra help in the last few days. This allows for primary caregivers to take breaks, which is critical. They need extra people available or stopping by frequently to make sure that they have food and can rest, because it's easy to stop taking care of yourself when you are so focused on the patient. Families will require extra help staying on top of the details of their regular lives. They may need someone to walk the dog or do errands.

Sometimes families and friends have a large group around all the time, which is called sitting vigil. This can be a joyful time, with people laughing and sharing stories. But it can also be a hard time, because no one knows how long this final phase in someone's life will last. Vicki often tells patients and family members that this stage of the illness is more like a marathon than a sprint. There is still tremendous uncertainty. Be aware that you can always ask questions of hospice nurses about how events might unfold day to day. Caregivers should take the time to eat, rest, go for walks, and pace themselves.

Some people ask whether it's okay to die at home when children are present. There isn't a lot of data to guide us on this. Doctors often recommend that the dying patient stay in a space that affords some privacy so they can have quiet when they need it and so that children can have space to play and be kids but can still interact with the person who is dying as much as they want to or need to.

What If I Don't Want to Prolong My Dying?

Of course, people want to live longer when they are living with illness. And yet when they are in the last hours or days of life, most people don't want to prolong the experience of dying. To best serve the patient, medical professionals use an ethical principle called patient autonomy. It states that patients who are of sound mind, who are not confused or depressed, have the right to refuse treatments they don't want.

Many interventions can prolong the process of dying, and patients have the right to refuse them. They may choose to stop supplemental nutrition and hydration, antibiotics treating an infection, or blood thinners. I've had patients say to me, "Why can't we turn off my pacemaker so that I can die of my heart problems instead of the cancer?" The answer is that doctors can do that, and it is often a comfortable way to die. Any patient has the right to refuse treatment even if that treatment is life sustaining or life prolonging.

Patients sometimes choose not to take antibiotics for pneumonia in the final days of life. They do this because dying from pneumonia or any other infection can be very peaceful. People get drowsy as their blood pressure drops and drift away while sleeping. It can feel odd to talk about the final phase of life like this, but many people become practical and clear eyed about choosing a gentle death.

Some people don't have any medical interventions that they can refuse, because they don't have a growing infection or heart condition, but they can still make the decision to stop eating and drinking. Many people with advanced cancer aren't particularly interested in eating already, and they just stop pushing themselves to take in food and fluids. They keep their mouths moist with swabs but don't track their fluid intake and eventually become sleepier. This is a painless and gentle choice to make.

What Is Physician Aid in Dying?

In some states, doctors are allowed to assist patients who are critically ill and want to end their lives. As of this writing, it is legal in California, Colorado, Oregon, Washington, Montana, New Mexico, and Vermont. Each state has its own regulations, but they share several common features. The patient must be a resident of the state in which this is legal. More than one physician must certify that the patient has a terminal diagnosis and that the patient request is not made under duress or because of depression or untreated symptoms.

Typically the medication, which is usually a powerful barbiturate sedative, is prescribed only after a waiting period. Also, the patient must be able to take the medication without the assistance of another person.

The law in Oregon has been in effect since 1997, and we know that not all the patients who acquire the prescription actually use it. We also know that most who do use it are not doing so because of suffering from symptoms but because they want to have control over the timing of their death. Doctors have very mixed feelings about physician aid in dying. Some believe that it is a patient's right to make this decision, while for others it runs counter to every instinct they have about the role of medicine in our lives.

How Families Can Prepare

In the final days of life, people often experience new symptoms, including pain, shortness of breath or noisy breathing, and confusion. In the vast majority of cases, these can be well controlled with medication. If the patient isn't already on an opioid, he or she may need one at this time to manage pain and shortness of breath.

Haloperidol can help with confusion and delirium. Lorazepam will help with anxiety. There are also medications to treat the noisy breathing in the last hours of life, including atropine or hyoscyamine. Hospice providers often send a package of medications, called a comfort care kit, which contains many of these medications. Still, the job of any hospice care team is to actively manage these symptoms in the home and to be the eyes and ears of your oncology team. Make sure you call them if the symptoms are not being well controlled. If the hospice can't control these symptoms at home, the patient can still be admitted to an inpatient hospice facility or hospital to get stabilized, with the idea that the patient can return home once the symptoms have calmed down.

Family members sometimes ask whether they can give too much pain medication and accidentally kill the patient. As long as you are following the guidelines of the hospice nurse or a physician, you should be fine. If you have concerns about the amount of pain medication to give, call your hospice nurse for guidance. Sometimes the medical team will give enough pain medication to make patients comfortable even if they are sleepy or groggy much of the time as a result. The primary goal is to make sure that the patient continues to be comfortable and free of distress.

As people get closer to dying, their breathing pattern often becomes quite erratic with quick bursts of respirations interspersed between long, slow, deep breaths and sometimes gaps in breathing of twenty seconds or more. This is called Cheyne-Stokes respiration, and it usually means that people are actively dying. If this breathing pattern starts and your hospice nurse isn't present, then you should call the nurse, who will want to know. Sometimes the patient's breathing can sound coarse and noisy, but you don't need to panic. This is a normal part of the dying process. All human beings go through it. Vicki always tells the family to look at the person's face. If the brow looks furrowed or the person looks restless, then more medication may be needed to ease the breathing. If the person looks comfortable and the breathing is just noisy, then everything is okay.

Family Unity

I grew up in a large extended family, and one of my uncles was a priest who worked as a hospital chaplain. Early in my career as an oncologist, I asked him, "What was the most amazing thing you learned in your work helping dying patients?" He told me that, when people are dying, they become even more exaggerated forms of their true selves. What he meant was that if people are kind and gentle at heart, they become even more so as they are dying. If people are ornery at heart, they become even more so as they are dying. And, he said, the same is often true for the family who has to care for the dying patient. The stress of dying for both the patient and family is enormous, and family discord can lead to a bad death even if the symptoms are well controlled and there is a lot of extra help at home.

I had a patient named Gerry who was dying from metastatic colon cancer that developed after he had struggled for two decades with ulcerative colitis. Gerry's mother had been able to compel him to get an annual colonoscopy when he was in his twenties, but Gerry's wife, Lily, had no luck urging him to go for his screenings after their wedding. Unfortunately, when his cancer was detected, it was already metastatic. Gerry's mother blamed Lily for not making him get his annual screenings, and the two of them could hardly stand to be in the same room together.

Believe me, your medical team knows when two members of a family are carrying out a long-standing feud or when family members are bickering and taking sides over treatment decisions. Nurses in particular have a sixth sense for this, and they worry about patients going home to die in an environment filled with friction.

Sometimes, families can put their differences aside for the good of the patient. Other times, they can't, and this puts the patient at risk of having a bad death. In these cases, it is best for everyone if the care is delivered in a setting other than home.

Being Present at the Moment of Death

Family members also ask how to prepare for the moment of death. These questions come in lots of forms. Some ask whether the patient is afraid to leave the family, or they wonder whether they need to offer reassurances that it's okay to go. Many dying patients can still hear what is said to them even when they are no longer responding. It can be helpful to continue to talk to the person who is dying as though he or she can hear you. I've heard Vicki encourage loved ones to say whatever they feel comfortable communicating to the patient. That might include reassurances that it will be okay if they go and that you love them.

Some family members do want to travel to sit vigil or to say good-bye as death approaches. If family members feel that they want to see the patient one last time, you can encourage them to come and sit vigil. They should make plans knowing that they might not be able to be there at the moment of death. As an alternative, they can call and say what they have to say to the patient, even if the patient can't respond. Or they can compose a message that someone sitting with the patient can read aloud. The important thing is to communicate what you want to the patient.

Some people want to be present at the moment of their loved one's death. While the idea of being present at death can seem significant, it's not always possible. Many times, I've seen patients hang on and die only after some significant family member arrives to see them. It's as though they were waiting. And these stories are the ones that get repeated to friends. But patients don't always wait for family members to arrive. They also sometimes die while family members are using the bathroom or out getting coffee or sleeping. What I've learned is that the person who is dying seems to do this in his or her own way, and none of us can control when the moment of death will arrive.

Vicki often tells the story of her mother's death in Wisconsin. Vicki flew out from Boston to be with her mother during her final hours, but the cab driver got lost on the way from the airport to the nursing facility. When Vicki told the driver that she was going to see her dying mother, the cab driver started talking about his wife, who had died six months before. The more he talked, the more flustered and lost he became. Eventually, she arrived at her mother's side just a few minutes after her death. Vicki says that while being with her mother again was important to her, she understood that nothing could negate the love that she had for her mother or all of the ways she had worked to show her love over the years.

How Do I Know That Someone Has Died?

Doctors look for several signs that indicate that the patient has died. First, we touch the patient and look for a response. Next, we observe the person's breathing. This is a bit tricky in patients in the final hours of life because there may be pauses of a minute between breaths at the very end. These are the signs most families look for at home. When a clinician comes to verify the death, he or she will listen with a stethoscope to make sure that there are no heart sounds and examine the patient's eyes. When people die, their pupils don't respond to light, and they become fixed in a dilated, or open, state.

If you are sitting with a loved one, you might first notice that they are not responding to you. And then you'll watch for a minute or so and see no breathing movements. Also, don't be surprised if the skin has turned pale and bluish in the extremities and becomes cold to the touch or if the patient has become incontinent of urine or stool. I tell families to expect that everything will relax as the person dies. When you notice these signs, the next step is to call your hospice nurse if he or she is not already at your home. The hospice nurse will verify that the person has died. Once the hospice nurse has verified the death, he or she will likely wash the person's body and remove any medical equipment such as IVs or oxygen lines. Families can choose to be present for this care and even participate if they would like. That may sound strange, but some families find it a meaningful way to pay their final respects.

The nurse will then call either the patient's oncologist, palliative care physician, or hospice doctor to sign the death certificate. You can then call the funeral director, who will send someone to your home to remove your loved one in a stretcher. If someone dies and is not enrolled in hospice, an ambulance is required by law in many states to bring a patient to the hospital to be pronounced dead. That's one of the many reasons why doctors advise patients to enroll in hospice.

Bereavement

The hours and days immediately following a person's death are typically busy. Family members may have services to prepare for, and there are guests who come to pay their respects. This is an emotional time that can often pass in a blur. And then friends and more distant relatives go back to their regular lives. Loved ones tell me that this is the hardest part. They ask themselves, "What now?"

The bereavement period is always one of firsts. First meals without someone, the first holidays, the first family vacation, the first time you want to call the person only to realize you can't. These are hard. Some memories are comforting, while others are painful. Vicki often tells people that it's hard to know how you will feel at any given point in grieving. Sometimes your friends think you should be sad, and you will feel okay. Other times, your friends will think you should be getting back into the rhythm of your life, and instead you feel like you've been hit by a truck and all you can do is cry all day. These feelings are all normal. It's important to be kind to yourself throughout this process.

Sometimes you might need additional support during the grieving process. Every hospice offers bereavement support services. This might be in the form of support groups or individual short-term counseling. You can take part in these services even if your loved one wasn't enrolled in hospice. Any hospice that receives federal support is required to provide bereavement services to anyone in its area.

In the weeks and months that follow someone's death, you may find that you still have the opportunity to be in a relationship with the person who has died. It's a very different kind of relationship, but it's still there. Often families will tell me, "I know what Mom would think about this. It sounds crazy, but I still feel like I can have a conversation with her."

It's also normal to have questions for the clinical care team about the patients' care after they have died. Vicki and I, like most clinicians, are happy to talk to loved ones after the death of a patient. Sometimes we do this to answer questions, and sometimes it is just to check in and say a final good-bye. I always call the family after one of my patients has died. I know how hard families work to support a patient during cancer care. Often close family members need someone to talk to about what their loved one experienced during the final days and hours before death. Sometimes, a member of the clinical team is the only person with whom you feel you can share these details. Cancer treatment can bring doctors, nurses, patients, and families close together. We like the opportunity to check in as well and to express to family members what was special about the patient.

A Final Note

VICKI AND I HOPE THAT this book can be a resource and a comfort for patients at every stage of cancer. It is our hope that this book empowers readers to ask important questions of their doctors and to engage with their care team in a meaningful way. We also want to demonstrate what care can be like when oncology and palliative care work together, because these two disciplines together can do more for patients than either can do alone. As an oncologist working closely with Vicki, I've learned that integrating palliative care and cancer treatment helps patients to better understand their diagnosis and to better manage their symptoms throughout treatment so that they can live as well as they can for as long as they can.

What we hope has shone through in these pages is that Vicki and I feel honored to do this work. We get to witness the courage of patients and families as they endeavor to live fully despite an uncertain future. It is enormously rewarding and humbling to care for patients with cancer. We have learned so much from our patients, who have been extraordinarily generous to us by sharing their insights but also by allowing us to see their strength, creativity, and humor while facing this difficult diagnosis. Vicki and I are better parents, spouses, and physicians because of our relationships with our patients. They have taught us everything we needed to know to write this book.

INDEX

abscess, 202, 210

absolute neutrophil count (ANC), 82, 204

acetaminophen (Tylenol), 52, 67, 157, 160, 161, 203

acupuncture, 75

acute decline, 308–10

acute lymphocytic leukemia (ALL), 46, 49

acute myelogenous leukemia (AML), 46, 47, 49

adenocarcinoma, 19, 31

adjuvant treatment, 38–41, 58

adrenal insufficiency, 227

advance health directives, 282–83, 306

advancing cancer, 41, 257–80; acute decline, 308–10; asking oncologist what they would do in patient's situation, 302; being in denial, 273–74, 277; best- and worst-case scenarios, 260–61; clinical trials, 267–70; coping with getting down, 279–80; doctor's reluctance to discuss death, 275; entering new phase of treatment, 258–59; family meetings about, 270; giving up hope, 274–75; how much time you have left, 276–77, 304, 308; how much you want to know, 275–76; practical concerns, 281–92; prognostic awareness, 272–74, 277, 306; resistance to targeted therapy, 259–60; slow decline, 305–7; subacute decline, 307–8; supportive care, 25, 26, 48, 75, 296, 297, 302; symptom management, 261–67; treatment options, 267; what you want to know, 275–78; when chemotherapy is no longer effective, 293–302

advocating for yourself, 5, 116, 282

aggressive treatment, 23, 24, 44; breast cancer, 290; colon cancer, 216; hematologic cancers, 46, 47, 53, 54, 307; lung cancer, 237; for pain, 158, 162, 168, 227–28; pancreatic cancer, 36

alanine aminotransferase (ALT), 86

alkaline phosphatase (ALP), 85

ALL (acute lymphocytic leukemia), 46, 49

allergies: blood products, 222, 266; chemotherapy, 71–72; IV contrast, 90; medications, 16

Aloxi (palonosetron), 126, 141

ALP (alkaline phosphatase), 85

ALT (alanine aminotransferase), 86

alternative therapies, 104, 197–98, 267, 299

Ambien, 230

American Society of Clinical Oncology, 6

amitriptyline, 241

AML (acute myelogenous leukemia), 46, 47, 49

analgesics. See pain management

anaphylaxis, 71, 90

ANC (absolute neutrophil count), 82, 204

clinical trials, 7, 25, 106, 209, 258, 297, 306, 309; adjuvant therapy, 39, 58; chemotherapy, 26, 260, 267, 269, 301; colon cancer, 26; drugs for anorexia-cachexia, 185; at end of life, 286; experimental drugs, 296–97, 298, 302; informed consent for participation, 268–70; oral blood thinners, 178, 213; in other countries, 298–99; phase I, II, and III, 267–68; proton beam radiation, 61

CLL (chronic lymphocytic leukemia), 46, 49, 307

Clostridium difficile colitis, 152

CML (chronic myelogenous leukemia), 46, 49

codeine, 181

cognitive behavioral therapy (CBT), 135, 174, 181–82

cognitive impairment, 247–54. *See also* confusion

Colace (docusate), 147, 148

colon, 137, 138, 144; effects of constipation, 140–41, 144, 145–46; immunotherapy attacking, 63, 207; obstruction, 123, 145–46

colon cancer, 15, 19, 46, 151; adjuvant chemotherapy, 40–41; bleeding, 83, 216–17, 219, 220; dying from, 309, 327; fatigue and, 232, 266, 296; metastatic, 24, 33, 89, 96, 143, 180, 220, 266, 296, 309, 327; ostomy bag and sexuality, 117; pain medication, 180–81; pulmonary embolus, 213; survival rates, 37, 39–41; treatment options, 24, 26, 296

colonoscopy, 63, 141, 149, 219, 327

colostomy, 146

Compazine (prochlorperazine), 126, 129, 130

complete blood count (CBC), 69, 81, 82, 204

computed tomography (CT), 52, 87, 88, 89–91, 144, 201, 262, 264; abdominal, 218, 220; in advancing cancer, 278, 296, 315; bile duct, 85, 86; chest, 174, 175, 176, 177, 179, 209, 214; IV contrast for,

90; vs. MRI, 92, 251; PET-CT scan, 45, 91; radiation dose, 59, 93; reading scans, 90–91

confusion, 28, 247–50, 289; brain metastases and, 251, 310; causes, 249; delirium, 250; at end of life, 320, 322, 325–26; infection and, 201; medication-induced, 135, 192, 246, 249; spacing out, 251

consciousness, loss of, 248

constipation, 3, 136–37, 260; abdominal tumors and, 133, 145–46, 264; cycling between diarrhea and, 139, 150–51; dehydration and, 144; diet and, 137, 190; false feeling of, 144–47; hypercalcemia and, 146–47; nausea due to, 123, 124, 126, 131, 132; signs of, 139–41; treatment, 147–50; weight loss and, 186

constipation, medication-induced, 141–44; antacids, 141, 143; blood pressure drugs, 141, 143–44; 5HT3 antagonists, 126, 141, 142–43, 149; opioids, 130–31, 141, 142, 149, 150, 167; tricyclic antidepressants, 241

Conversation Project, 285–86

coping, 2, 7, 96–110; asking why, 97–98; with body changes, 111–19; vs. fighting, 98–99; with getting down, 279–80; with other people, 106–10; strategies, 100–104; symptom management, 99–100; talk therapy, 238–40, 242

coughing: anaphylaxis and, 71; of blood, 28, 214, 218; infection and, 200, 201, 203, 205, 209–10; lung cancer and, 252; pneumonitis and, 61; swallowing difficulty and, 188; vomiting and, 132–33

cough medicine, 181

creatinine, 85

cremation, 289–90

crizotinib, 252, 253, 259

CT. *See* computed tomography

curability, 34–35, 44–45; adjuvant chemotherapy and, 39–41; best- and worst-case scenarios, 35–36, 260–61; chemo holidays and, 76;

curability (*continued*)
    incurable cancers, 8, 20, 23, 24, 34, 42, 44, 45, 257, 259, 271, 293, 300, 302, 315; liquid tumors, 46–48, 53; recurrence and, 38; staging and, 22–23, 44, 53
Cymbalta (duloxetine), 241
cytokines, 194

Decadron. *See* dexamethasone
deconditioning, 73, 173, 175–76, 231
dehydration, 85, 130; constipation due to, 140, 141, 142, 144, 147, 151; due to diarrhea, 153, 299; fatigue and, 229, 233; hypercalcemia and, 147; opioid-induced, 142
delirium, 250–51, 289, 319, 320, 326
denial, 273–74, 277
depression, 105, 235–40, 248–49, 324, 325; after bone marrow transplant, 54; fatigue and, 224, 231; hope and, 274, 275; palliative care and, 6, 54, 239; vs. sadness, 236–38, 279; sleep problems and, 231, 236; steroid-induced, 193; symptoms, 236; talk therapy for, 238–40; treatment, 186, 231, 239, 240–41; weight loss and, 186
dexamethasone (Decadron): for brain swelling, 253; infection risk and, 82; insomnia due to, 130; for nausea, 126, 127, 227; to stimulate appetite and energy, 193, 233–34
diagnosis, 19; confirmation, 14, 15; emotional reactions, 1–3, 13, 15; tests, 1, 8–9, 14, 17, 21
diarrhea, 8, 9, 150–54, 299; causes, 152; chemotherapy-induced, 73, 136, 137, 151, 152, 238, 302; cycling between constipation and, 139, 150–51; depression and, 238; diet and, 73, 97, 137, 148; due to lactose intolerance, 189; immunotherapy-induced, 63; IV contrast–induced, 90; laxatives and, 149–50; radiation-induced, 60; SSRI-induced, 241; treatment, 152–54

diet/nutrition: artificial nutrition, 194–96; calorie intake, 189–90, 194; constipation and, 137, 147, 190; diarrhea due to, 73, 97, 137; energy drink supplements, 190; fiber in, 137, 142, 147, 148, 190; lactose intolerance, 185, 189; mucositis and, 187; nutritional supplements, 197–99; pancreatic insufficiency and, 188; strategies to keep weight on, 189–90. *See also* eating
Dilaudid (hydromorphone), 130, 150, 162, 169, 182, 262
diltiazem, 184
diphenhydramine (Benadryl), 187, 228
diphenoxylate, 153
distraction strategy, 100, 101, 242
dizziness, 123, 319, 320
DNA, 20, 32, 47, 57, 62, 63; tests, 43, 50, 94
docusate (Colace), 147, 148
dopamine antagonists, 126, 129, 130
doxepin, 241
driving, 78, 168
dronabinol (Marinol), 192, 311
Dulcolax (bisacodyl), 147, 149
duloxetine (Cymbalta), 241
dying and death, 105, 303–31; acknowledging possibility of, 273, 274, 307; after acute decline, 308–10; adjuvant chemotherapy to reduce risk, 40–41; from arrhythmia, 285; being in denial about, 273–74, 277; bereavement, 330–31; from blood clots or bleeding, 215; breathing pattern during, 326, 329; with children present, 324; choosing a health care proxy, 77, 282, 283, 322; communicating with family/friends about, 314–17; decision not to prolong dying process, 324–25; discussing how you will die, 304–5; doctor's reluctance to discuss, 275; eating, drinking and, 311–12; end of life care, 285–87; family needs during,

319–21, 323–24; family preparation for, 325–26; family presence at moment of death, 327–29; family unity and, 327; in first year after diagnosis, 36; funerals and obituaries, 289–90; good death, 318; hearing during, 328; at home, 308, 319–21, 324; hospice care for, 288, 304, 310–11, 319–22; in ICU, 284, 309, 322–23; from infection, 210–11, 303, 324; in inpatient hospice, 322; knowing how much time you have left, 276–77, 304, 308; knowing when death has occurred, 329; vs. living with cancer, 312–13; MOLST and POLST forms, 282–84; patient's wishes related to, 318; physician aid in, 325; prognostic awareness of, 272–74, 277, 306; questions about process of, 303, 304–6; at residential hospice, 321–22; resuscitation and, 283–84, 286–87, 323; shortness of breath and, 182–83; after slow decline, 305–7; after subacute decline, 307–8; from treatment, 27; treatment goal of extending life by any amount, 301–2; what you want to know, 275–78

dysphagia. *See* swallowing difficulty

eating: avoiding guilt about, 190–92; effects of changes in smell and taste, 185, 186, 189; at end of life, 305, 311–12; fatigue and, 229; strategies in advancing cancer, 264–65; strategies to keep weight on, 189–90; swallowing difficulty, 74, 185–88, 195. *See also* appetite loss; diet/nutrition
echocardiogram, 174
Effexor XR (venlafaxine), 241
electrolytes, 84–85
embolization, 84, 216, 221
Emend (aprepitant), 126, 128
emergencies, oncologic, 27–28
emotional concerns, 3, 7, 10, 13, 15

end of life care, 285–87. *See also* dying and death
endoscopic retrograde pancreatico-duodenoscopy, 86
enemas, 148, 198, 299
energy bank account, 224
energy drink supplements, 190
enoxaparin, 178
enteral nutrition, 194
erectile dysfunction, 62, 117–18
erlotinib, 152, 301–2
erythromycin, 131, 186
erythropoietin, 178, 221
escitalopram (Lexapro), 241
esophagogastroscopy, 219
esophagus, 83, 131, 137, 138; bleeding in, 83, 219–20; cancer, 5, 79, 187, 188, 195, 220, 251, 260, 264, 277; yeast infection, 132
estrogen, 62, 118
exercise, 100, 225–26, 254, 259; aerobic, 231–32; cognitive, 249; effects of deconditioning, 73, 173, 175–76, 231; fatigue and, 231–32, 233; with G-tube, 11; neuropathy and, 113; pain and, 159; recommendations, 231–32; shortness of breath and, 173, 176, 178
experimental treatments, 25, 26, 267, 286, 298–302. *See also* clinical trials

family/friends, 106–10; asking for help, 109; bereavement, 330–31; blogs and websites for, 110; chemotherapy effects on, 76–78; communications about imminent death, 314–17; extended family and community, 109–10; family meetings, 270; family presence at moment of death, 327–29; having important conversations, 291; inner and outer orbits, 107–8, 314; managing relationships as cancer advances, 290–91; needs during patient's dying process, 319–21, 323–24; preparation for patient's death, 325–26; unity of, 327; writing letters to, 292, 314–17 fatigue, 10, 45, 157, 203, 223–34, 247, 249; in advancing cancer, 258, 261, 266–67, 271, 272, 276, 286, 292, 296, 303, 305, 306, 307, 308, 310; anemia and, 81, 227; chemotherapy-induced, 70, 72, 73, 75, 80; coping with, 100, 101, 105; dexamethasone for, 193; energy bank account, 224; episodic, causes of, 226; episodic vs. ongoing, 224; maximizing energy, 225–26; medication-induced, 228–29; medications for, 232–34; ongoing, causes of, 226–32; pain and, 227–28; radiation-induced, 60; rating scale for, 224; sex and, 115, 117; sleep problems and, 224, 226, 229–33

febrile neutropenia, 28, 205

feeding tube, 113, 194, 195, 196

fentanyl, 130, 161–62, 262

fertility, 65, 76

fever, 28, 45, 80, 177, 200, 307; blood product allergy and, 222; infection and, 201, 203, 210

fiber, 137, 142, 147, 148, 190

fistulas, 216, 220, 221

5-fluorouracil, 151, 152

5HT3 antagonists, 126–27, 141, 142, 149

flow strategy, 100, 103–4

fluconazole, 187

fluoxetine (Prozac), 241

flushing, 8, 9

fosaprepitant (Emend for injection), 126

funerals, 289–90

fungal infections, 132–33, 186–87, 202–3, 207

gabapentin (Neurontin), 160, 228, 230

gag reflex, 132

gastrointestinal (GI) tract, 138; artificial nutrition, 194–96; bacteria in, 81; bleeding in, 28, 83, 215, 216, 218–20, 309; cancers, 5, 19, 24, 148, 188, 196, 315; function, 137; obstruction, 131, 264; radiation effects, 60; varices, 216, 219–20

gastroparesis, 131–32, 133, 186

gene mutations, 20, 32, 44; targeted therapy for, 252, 259, 260; testing for, 94–95

genotyping, 19, 20–21

Goodman, Ellen, 285

graft versus host disease, 54, 152, 208

graft versus leukemia (or lymphoma) effect, 54

granisetron (Kytril), 126, 141, 142

gratitude, 100, 102, 280, 291, 314, 316

grief, 236, 284, 316

growth factor support, 82, 205

G-tube, 113, 114

hair loss, 62, 63, 72, 73–74, 108, 111–13, 114

headache, 148, 321; brain metastases and, 251, 260; nausea and, 124, 134; after spinal tap, 52

head and neck cancer, 19, 59, 215

health care proxy, 77, 282, 283, 322

heart attack, 62, 213

hematologic malignancies. See liquid tumors

hematopoiesis, 266

hemophilia, 218

hemorrhoids, 148, 216–17

hepatitis B, 222

hepatitis C, 222

hepatocellular cancer, 132

herbal remedies, 198

HER2 targeted therapy, 64, 260

history, medical, 13, 14, 15, 16–17

HIV infection, 82, 222

hope, 13, 16, 45, 106, 258, 269, 272; giving up, 236, 274–75, 300; for good death, 318

hormonal therapy, 61, 62, 118, 205, 305

hormone-sensitive cancers, 118

hormones in GI tract, 137, 145

hospice care, 36, 274, 276, 278, 287–89, 299, 303–4, 306; bereavement services, 330; choosing, 287; cost/payment for, 287, 289,

321; goal of, 288; home, 296, 308, 309, 310–11, 316; home, dying during, 319–30; ICD and, 285; inpatient, 288–89, 304, 306, 313, 326; inpatient, dying during, 322; "open access," 287; residential, dying during, 321–22; symptom management in final days, 326; verifying death has occurred, 329; when to enroll, 288

humor, 100, 102, 103, 108, 300, 334

hydromorphone (Dilaudid), 130, 150, 162, 169, 182, 262

hypercalcemia, 85, 145, 146–47

hypothyroidism, 145, 227

ibuprofen, 157, 159, 161

ICD (implantable cardiac defibrillator), 284–85

ICU (intensive care unit), dying in, 284, 309, 322–23

ileostomy, 146

imatinib, 24

immune system, 62–63, 81, 82, 84, 204, 222; bone marrow transplantation and, 207–8; chemotherapy effects, 200; fungal infections and, 203; how cancer spreads, 32; pneumonitis and, 176; steroid effects, 176

immunohistochemistry, 19, 20

immunotherapy, 8, 61, 62–63, 201, 206–7, 295; steroids and, 176–77

Imodium (loperamide), 73, 153, 154

implantable cardiac defibrillator (ICD), 284–85

infection(s), 10, 80, 200–211; antibiotic-resistant, 42, 64, 210, 259; blood tests and, 204; bone marrow failure and, 265–66; after bone marrow transplant, 207–8; from cancer, 208–9; closed space, 210; death from, 210–11, 303, 324; delirium due to, 250; dental procedures and, 204; diarrhea due to, 152; fatigue due to, 227, 230; fungal, 132–33, 186–87, 202–3, 207; herpes, 74, 187, 203; HIV, 82, 222; immune defense

against, 51, 81–83, 200, 204; immunotherapy-related, 206–7; intrathecal pump and, 263; management as cancer progresses, 209–10, 257, 258, 261, 323, 324; mouth, 186–87; nausea due to, 123, 124, 132–33; neutropenia and, 204–5; new symptoms and, 201–2; opportunistic, 82; pneumonia, 132, 173, 174, 175, 177, 209–10, 324; of portacath, 68–69; risk after chemotherapy, 202; risk from blood transfusion, 221–22; risk of catching, 203–4; sex and risk of, 116–17; signs of, 201; steroid-related, 82–83, 132, 186, 203; TPN and, 196; treatment-induced, 206; treatment of, 202–3; urinary tract, 42, 201, 202, 259; viral, 82, 187, 202, 203, 208

inflammation: brain, 252, 253; GI tract, 124; liver, 86; lung, 60, 173, 175, 176–77; NSAIDs for, 159–60; radiation-induced, 60

informed consent, 301; for clinical trial participation, 268–70

insomnia. See sleep problems

intellectualization, 100, 104

intensive care unit (ICU), dying in, 284, 309, 322–23

Internet research, 2, 34, 107

intubation, 83, 284

irinotecan, 73, 151, 152

job, treatment scheduling and, 4, 9

joy, 100, 102, 114, 225, 279, 286, 314, 316

Kaopectate, 187

kidney: cancer, 175; dysfunction, 90, 92, 144, 323; function tests, 84, 85; NSAID effects, 160

Kytril (granisetron), 126, 141, 142

lactose intolerance, 185, 189

lactulose, 147, 149

lapatinib, 152

laughter, 16, 103, 312, 313, 319, 323

infections after bone marrow transplant for, 207–8; low lymphocyte count and infections in, 82; pathologic diagnosis, 52–53; scans in, 44, 51, 91

magic mouthwash, 187
magnesium, blood level, 84
magnesium citrate, 147, 149
magnetic resonance imaging (MRI), 9, 52, 87, 88, 92, 250; brain, 51, 92, 248, 251, 252, 253, 260; vs. CT, 92, 251; reading scans, 92
MAO-I (monoamine oxidase inhibitor), 241
marginally effective drugs, 297
marijuana, medical, 197
Marinol (dronabinol), 192, 311
massage therapy, 75, 299
mastectomy, 95, 111, 113, 115
MDS (myelodysplastic syndrome), 48, 93, 265
Medical Orders for Life Sustaining Treatment (MOLST), 282–84
Medicare, 289
meditation, 98, 100, 103, 242, 259
megestrol acetate (Megace), 192, 311
melanoma, 19, 245, 265, 307; brain metastasis, 214, 251; immuno-therapy, 63, 176; with pulmonary embolus, 214
melatonin, 230
memory impairment, 249
Metamucil, 147, 148
metastases, 18, 21, 258, 271; abdominal/pelvic, 133, 145; bone, 25, 58, 89, 106, 146, 158, 167, 170; brain, 28, 92, 124, 134, 214, 221, 248–49, 251–53, 260, 310; liver, 9, 23, 31, 32, 33, 41, 140, 251, 260, 272, 307–8, 319; lung, 32, 93, 173, 180, 307, 315; lymph node, 58, 220; on MRI, 92; radiation therapy for, 58; spinal, 170, 202; staging and, 33–34, 41
methadone, 161, 162–63
methylnaltrexone (Relistor), 150
methylphenidate (Ritalin), 167, 229, 232–33, 249

metoclopramide (Reglan), 126, 131, 133, 186
metoprolol, 184
Milk of Magnesia, 143, 147, 149
Miralax (polyethylene glycol), 143, 147, 149, 151
mirtazapine (Remeron), 186, 193, 230, 241
modafinil, 232
molecular pathology, 19, 20–21, 44, 63, 95, 252
MOLST (Medical Orders for Life Sustaining Treatment), 282–84
monoamine oxidase inhibitors (MAO-I), 241
morphine, 92, 130, 150, 158, 160, 161–62, 165, 180, 182, 229, 309
mouth: dry, 124, 241; sores, 66, 72, 74, 124, 186–87; yeast infection, 124, 186–87
mouthwashes, 187
MRI. *See* magnetic resonance imaging
mucositis, 74, 185–87
music therapy, 75
Mycelex mouthwash, 187
myelodysplastic syndrome (MDS), 48, 93, 265
myeloid cells, 81
myeloma, 43
myelophthisis, 266

naloxone, 147, 150
napping, 60, 230
Nardil (phenelzine), 241
National Cancer Institute of Canada, 301
National Comprehensive Cancer Network (NCCN), 42, 223
nausea/vomiting, 3, 7, 123–35, 286, 305, 322; abdominal tumors and, 133, 264; anticipatory, 124, 129; anxiety and, 124, 135; break-through, 129; chemotherapy-induced, 5, 62, 71, 72, 75, 100, 125–30, 151; doctor's questions about, 124; drug-induced, 125; due to constipation, 123, 124, 126, 131, 132; due to upper airway irritation, 132–33; gastroparesis

nausea/vomiting (*continued*)
and, 131–32; liver dysfunction
and, 133–34; marijuana for, 197;
mood effects, 238; neurologic
causes, 134; opioid-induced,
130–31, 167; radiation-induced,
60; sensory causes, 134–35;
staying ahead of, 129–30; triggers, 123–24; venting G-tube for,
265; VOMITING mnemonic for
causes of, 123–24; weight loss
due to, 185, 186, 191. *See also*
antiemetics

NCCN (National Comprehensive
Cancer Network), 42, 223

neoadjuvant therapy, 38, 58

nerve blocks, 170–71

Neulasta, 82

Neupogen, 82

neuroendocrine tumors, 9, 152, 154

Neurontin (gabapentin), 160, 228,
230

neuropathy, 5, 74, 99, 111, 113, 279;
treatment, 160, 228, 241

neutropenia, 28, 204–5

neutrophils, 81–82, 200, 204, 205

nivolomab, 152

NK-1 receptor antagonists, 126,
127–28

nonsteroidal anti-inflammatory
drugs (NSAIDs), 159–60

nortriptyline (Pamelor), 241

nosebleeds, 217

NSAIDs (nonsteroidal anti-
inflammatory drugs), 159–60

nurse practitioners, 3, 6, 28, 29, 69,
144, 150, 151, 204, 261

obituary, 290

octreotide, 9, 153, 154

odynophagia, 186–87

olanzapine (Zyprexa), 135, 182, 192,
230, 241, 246

Ommaya reservoir, 253

oncologists, 2–10; asking what they
would do in patient's situation,
302; family meetings with, 77–78;
first meeting with, 13–20;
selection, 28–29

oncology, 4, 8

ondansetron (Zofran), 71, 126, 141,
142–43, 151

opioid antagonists, 150

opioids: constipation due to,
130–31, 141, 142, 149, 150, 167;
discontinuation, 169; driving
and, 168; fear of addiction, 155,
168, 180; intrathecal, 170, 263;
IV infusion, 169; long-acting,
161–62, 228–29; long-acting plus
short-acting, 164–66; loss of
effectiveness over time, 169;
before MRI, 92; nausea induced
by, 130–31, 167; patient-controlled
analgesia, 169–70, 182–183;
rotation of, 262; sedative effects,
228–29; short-acting, 160–61,
228–29; for shortness of breath,
180–81; side effects, 167; timing
administration of, 163–64;
tolerance to, 262–63. *See also*
specific drugs

optimism, 27, 98, 100, 101–2, 239,
242–44, 272

osteoporosis, 62, 193

ostomies, 112, 113, 117, 146

ovarian cancer, 75, 94, 114, 196,
271–72, 277

oxycodone (Oxycontin), 67, 130,
140, 150, 158, 159, 160, 161, 162,
169, 262

oxygenation, 81, 172–78, 212, 283

oxygen therapy, 180, 182, 284, 287

paclitaxel, 5, 179

pain, 17, 155–59; abdominal, 124,
133, 140–41, 258; anxiety and,
155, 168, 246; back, 28; breakthrough, 164–65, 262; after
chemotherapy, 70; chest, 28, 178,
309; coping with, 5, 7; describing
intensity of, 156–59; fatigue and,
227–28; intermittent, 161; of
mouth sores, 74, 186–87; neck, 89;
neuropathic, 113; of pleurodesis,
179; referred, 228; sleep and, 25,
155, 156, 158, 230, 262; during
swallowing, 186–87

pain management, 3, 99, 155–71; in
advancing cancer, 262–63, 276;